SUGAR FREE . . . SWEETS AND TREATS

By Judith Soley Majors

Apple Press
Milwaukie, Oregon

First Printing

Printed in the United States of America

Library of Congress Catalog Card Number: 82-073049

ISBN: 0-9602238-6-X

Published by: Apple Press
5536 S.E. Harlow
Milwaukie, Oregon 97222

American Diabetes Association, Inc
OREGON AFFILIATE, INC.

3607 S.W. Corbett Portland, Oregon 97201 (503) 228-0849

June 30, 1982

"Sugar Free...Sweets and Treats"

With the blessing and the approval
of the
Dietetic Committee
American Diabetes Association, Inc.
Oregon Affiliate, Inc.

Rita Dewart
Executive Director

Rita Dewart

To “Mom”,

Leora Soley, who patiently taught me to cook and encouraged creativity and experimentation – never complaining about the mess!

And to “Dad”,

Al Soley who courageously tried everything I cooked!

*In memory of Barbara Verhoff Billette, RD who cared and shared her knowledge and talents bringing sunshine into the lives of others.

With very special heartfelt thanks:
Jack and Carrie, my husband and daughter, never ending love and support
American Diabetes Association, Inc; Oregon Affiliate, Inc., technical assistance
My friends, recipe sharing, testing and helpful suggestions
Vicky Hutchinson, encouragement and assistance
Clarence and Annie Billette, sharing time with Barbara.

EXCHANGE PROGRAM

The exchange program offers a variety of food to fit each individual likes and needs in specific amounts. By using the six exchange lists and foods in specified numbers and amounts to fit your diet, you can create a variety of taste sensations and almost forget you're on a diet!

The exchange program is simply a trade of one food for another in a specific food group for a food that is nearly equal in calories, carbohydrates, protein and fat. Also foods in each exchange group have similar mineral and vitamin content.

A well balanced diet consists of foods from each food group, as no single exchange group can supply all the nutrients our body requires for good health.

The energy value of food is expressed by the calorie count. The primary energy sources are fats, proteins and carbohydrates. Sugars and starches are the most common carbohydrates. The foods in the following exchange lists work together to provide the necessary nutrients that are essential to body function.

The real trick is to carefully measure the amounts of food used. All amounts are given in household measurement and are based on the "new" ADA exchange lists.

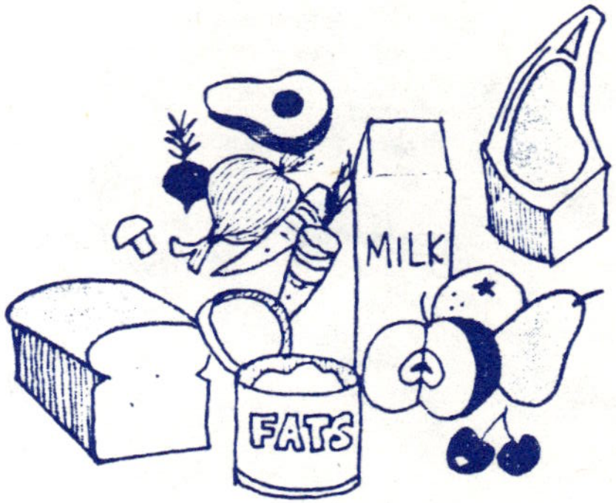

BASIC EXCHANGE LIST

FREE EXCHANGES

These foods and seasonings contain negligible amounts of protein, fat or carbohydrate and may be used in unlimited amounts.

- Diet type (calorie free) beverages
- Coffee
- Horseradish
- Unsweetened pickles
- Raw lettuce
- Unsweetened gelatin
- Salt and pepper
- Garlic
- Celery salt
- Radishes
- Lemon juice
- Tea
- Lime juice
- Paprika
- Parsley
- Mustard
- Onion powder and salt
- Vinegar
- Cinnamon and Nutmeg
- Fat free bouillon
- Fat free consomme
- Unsweetened cranberries
- Mint
- Herbs
- Soy sauce
- Non-calorie sweeteners

MILK EXCHANGES

LIST 1

Non Fat– Low Fat and Whole Milk

Each milk exchange contains 12 grams of carbohydrate, 8 grams of protein, a neglible amount of fat and 80 calories.

NON FAT FORTIFIED MILK	
Skim or non-fat milk	1 cup
Powdered non-fat milk (dry)	⅓ cup
Canned evaporated skim milk	½ cup
Skim type buttermilk	1 cup
Unflavored yogurt (from skim milk)	1 cup
LOW FAT FORTIFIED MILK	
1% fat fortified milk (omit ½ fat exchange)	1 cup
2% fat fortified milk (omit 1 fat exchange)	1 cup
Unflavored yogurt from 2% fortified milk (omit 1 fat exchange)	1 cup
WHOLE MILK (omit 2 fat exchanges for each)	
Whole milk	1 cup
Evaporated canned whole milk	½ cup
Buttermilk made from whole milk	1 cup
Unflavored yogurt (made from whole milk)	1 cup
Ice milk	1 cup

Milk is the leading source of calcium. It also contains protein, phosphorus, B-vitamins, magnesium and vitamins A and D. The milk exchange may be used to drink or included in recipes or added to cereal, coffee or other foods as desired. Remember to count the amount of milk added to other foods.

LIST 2
VEGETABLE EXCHANGES

Each vegetable exchange contains approximately 5 grams of carbohydrate, 2 grams of protein and 25 calories.

*One exchange equals ½ cup unless noted.

Artichoke (1)	Chilies	Onions
Asparagus	Collards	Rhubarb
Bean Sprouts	Cucumber	Rutabagas
Beets	Dandelion	Sauerkraut
Broccoli	Egg Plant	Spinach
Brussel Sprouts	Green Beans (string)	Squash (summer)
Cabbage	Green Pepper	Tomatoes
Carrots	Kale	Tomato Juice
Cauliflower	Mushrooms	Turnips
Celery	Mustard Greens	V-8 Juice
Chard	Okra	Zucchini

The following vegetables may be used **raw** as desired. Calories negligible.

Alfalfa Sprouts
Chicory
Chinese Cabbage
Chives
Endive
Escarole
Lettuce
Onion Tops (green)
Parsley
Radishes
Watercress

*Check the bread exchange list for starchy vegetables.

Vegetables are rich sources of vitamins and fiber is present in all vegetables.

LIST 3
FRUIT EXCHANGES

Each fruit exchange contains 10 grams of carbohydrate and 40 calories.

Fruits may be used fresh, dried, cooked, frozen, canned or raw as long as there are no sugars added.

Fruit	**Amount**	**Fruit**	**Amount**
Apple	1 small	Grapes	12 large
Apple Juice	⅓ cup	Grape Juice	¼ cup
Applesauce (sugar free)	½ cup	Honeydew Melon	½ medium
Apricots (fresh or dried)	2(4 halves)	Mango	½ small
Banana	½ small	Nectarine	1 small
Berries:		Pear	1 small
Blackberries	½ cup	Orange Juice	½ cup
Blueberries	½ cup	Papaya	¾ cup
Cranberries (sugar free)	Free Ex.	Peach	1 medium
		Pear	1 small
Raspberries	½ cup	Pineapple	½ cup
Strawberries	¾ cup	Pineapple Juice	⅓ cup
Cantaloupe	¼ small	Plums	2 medium
Cherries	10 large	Pomegranate	1 small
Cider	⅓ cup	Prunes	2 medium
Dates	2	Prune Juice	¼ cup
Figs	1	Raisins	2 tbs.
Grapefruit	½	Tangelo	1 small
Grapefruit Juice	½ cup	Tangerine	1 medium

Fruits supply fiber, various amounts of vitamins A and C, folacin and potassium.

LIST 4

BREAD EXCHANGES

(Breads, cereals, crackers and starchy vegetables)

Each bread exchange contains 15 grams of carbohydrate, 2 grams of protein and 70 calories.

Breads	Amount	Crackers	Amount
Bagel	½ small	Arrow root	3
Pumpernickle	1 slice	Graham	2-2½" square
Rye Bread	1 slice	Oyster	20
Raisin	1 slice	Pretzels	25-3 ¼" long x ⅛" dia.
White (incl. French)	1 slice		
Whole wheat	1 slice	Rye Krisp	3
Popover	1	Saltines	6
English Muffin	½ small	Soda Crackers	4
Plain roll (bread type)	1		
Hot dog bun	½	Hamburger bun	½
Croutons	½ cup plain		
Dried bread crumbs	3 tbps		
Bread sticks	4-9" long		
Tortillas	1-6" dia.		

Cereals	Amount
All Bran	½ cup
Bran Flakes	½ cup
Other ready to eat unsweetened cereal	¾ cup
Puffed cereal (unsweetened)	1 cup
Cereal, cooked	½ cup
Grits, cooked	½ cup
Rice, cooked	½ cup
Barley, cooked	½ cup
Pasta, cooked (noodle products)	½ cup
Popcorn (popped without fat)	3 cups
Cornmeal	2 tablespoons
Flour	2-½ tablespoons
Wheat germ	¼ cup
Cornstarch	2 tablespoons

Miscellaneous Foods	Amount
Ice Cream (omit 2 fat exchanges)	½ cup
French Fries (omit 1 fat exchange)	8-3" x ½"
Potato Chips (omit 2 fat exchanges)	14
Corn chips (omit 2 fat exchanges)	15

Starchy Vegetables	Amount
Beans (dried and cooked)	½ cup
Peas (dried and cooked)	½ cup
Lentils (dried and cooked)	½ cup
Peas (green canned or frozen)	½ cup
Corn (canned or frozen)	⅓ cup
Corn on the cob	1 small
Lima beans	½ cup
Parsnips	⅔ cups
Potato (white)	1 small
Potato mashed	½ cup
Potato (sweet)	¼ cup
Pumpkin	¾ cup
Squash (winter)	½ cup
Yam	¼ cup

*Starchy vegetables are included in the bread exchange list as they contain the same amount of protein and carbohydrates as one slice of bread.

LIST 5

MEAT EXCHANGES

Meat is divided into three categories. Each LEAN MEAT exchange contains 7 grams of protein, 3 grams of fat and 55 calories. For each MEDIUM-FAT MEAT EXCHANGE count 75 calories and omit ½ fat exchange. For each HIGH-FAT MEAT EXCHANGE count 100 calories and omit 1 fat exchange.

Lean Meat (Fat Removed)	Amount
Beef: baby beef, chopped beef, chuck, flank steak, london broil, tenderloin plate, ribs, top and bottom round (steak and roast), all cuts rump, sirloin and tripe.	1 ounce
Lamb: Leg, rib, loin, shoulder and shank	1 ounce
Pork: Leg, rump, center shank, smoked ham (center slices)	1 ounce
Veal: Leg, loin, rib, cutlets	1 ounce
Poultry: Flesh only (skin removed), chicken, turkey, cornish game hen, pheasant	1 ounce
Seafoods and Fish: Any fresh or frozen fish	1 ounce
Canned salmon, tuna, mackeral, crab or lobster	¼ cup 1 ounce or
Clams, oysters, scallops, shrimp	5 medium
Sardines, drained	3
Cheese: Those containing less than 5% butterfat	1 ounce
Lean meat	
Cottage Cheese: Dry, 2% butterfat	¼ cup

*Check pre-basted and liquid cured meats and poultry for sugar and fat contents.

MEDIUM FAT MEAT EXCHANGES

Beef: Ground (15% fat) corned beef (canned), rib eye, ground round	1 ounce
Pork: Loin (all cuts, shoulder (picnic), Boston butt, broiled ham, canadian bacon	1 ounce
All: Liver, heart, kidney, sweetbreads	1 ounce
Cheese: Mozzarella, Ricotta, Farmer's Cheese,	1 ounce
Parmesan, grated	3 tbps
Eggs: Raw or cooked (no fat added)	1

HIGH FAT MEAT EXCHANGES

	Amount
Beef: Ground beef (more than 20% fat) corned beef brisket, brisket, commercial hamburger, chuck, rib roasts and steaks	1 ounce
Veal: Breast	1 ounce
Lamb: Breast	1 ounce
Pork: Spare ribs, loin, ground pork, sausage, country style ham, deviled ham	1 ounce
Poultry: Duck, goose	1 ounce
Cheese: Cheddar	1 ounce
Prepared Meats: Frankfurters, weiners	1 small
Cold cuts (4 ½" x ⅛" slice)	1

LIST 6

FAT EXCHANGES

Each fat exchange contains 5 grams of fat and 45 calories.

Saturated Fats	**Amounts**
Margarine (regular)	1 teaspoon
Butter	1 teaspoon
Bacon Grease	1 teaspoon
Bacon, cooked crisp	1 slice
Cream, light	2 tbps.
Cream, sour	2 tbps.
Cream, heavy	1 tbp.
Cream cheese	1 tbp
Mayonnaise	1 teaspoon
Salad dressing (mayonnaise type)	2 teaspoons
Lard	1 teaspoon

Polyunsaturated Fats	
Soft margarine (tub or stick)	1 teaspoon
Avocado	1/8-4" dia.
Corn Oil	1 teaspoon
Cottonseed Oil	1 teaspoon
Safflower Oil	1 teaspoon
Soy Oil	1 teaspoon
Sunflower Oil	1 teaspoon
Olive Oil	1 teaspoon
Peanut Oil	1 teaspoon
Olives	5 small
Nuts:	
Almonds	10 whole
Pecans	2 large
Spanish Peanuts	20 whole
Virginia Peanuts	10 whole
Walnuts	6 small
Other Nuts	6 small

Fats are concentrated calorie sources and should be measured carefully. The origin of fats is either animal or vegetable and they range from solid hard fats to liquid oils. Generally, vegetable fats (corn oil, peanut oil, etc.) remain liquid at room temperature. Saturated fat is often hard at room temperature and is primarily from animal food products (butter, bacon, meat fat, etc.).

Calculation key =

Exchanges are from the "New" American Diabetes Association Exchange Lists. These lists are included in the book.

C = grams of carbohydrate
P = grams of protein
F = grams of fat

*All values are given per serving unless otherwise specified.

Weights: 1 ounce or 30 grams

Volumes: 1 teaspoon or 5 milliliters
1 tablespoon or 15 milliliters
1 ounce or 30 milliliters
1 cup = 8 ounces or .24 liters or 240 milliliters

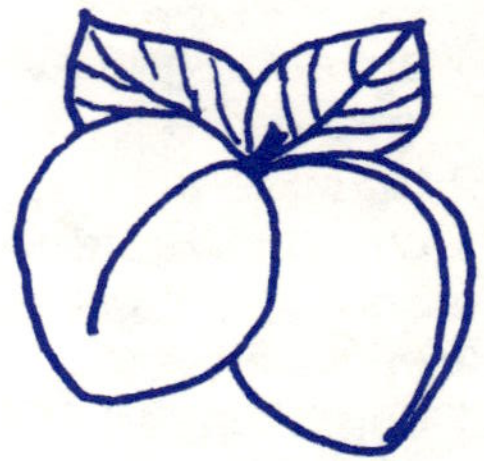

HELPFUL HINTS

Spices add a rich sweet flavor to fruit sweetened goodies. The "sweet" spices are cinnamon, nutmeg, cloves, allspice and ginger if mixed with another "sweet" spice. Vanilla and almond combined with spices blend the sweetness and enhance the flavor. These may be used to taste and exchanged within recipes to suit your taste. Spices should be used sparingly – just to enhance – not overwhelm natural flavors and sweetness.

Refrigerate or freeze (for later use) fruit sweetened baked goods. Fruit sweetened goodies do not have the preservative quality of sugared products and will spoil much more rapidly than their sugared counterparts.

Frozen unsweetened concentrates are a highly concentrated natural sweetener and provide much sweetness in small amounts. They can often be used to replace water or milk in a conventional recipe to add flavor and sweetness. I usually buy large cans (more economical and convenient) and scoop out the amount I need and replace the remainder in the freezer for later use. Concentrates can be combined for interesting flavor combinations.

When substituting fruit juice or concentrate in baked goods you must take into consideration the extra bulk, density and fiber. I find it necessary to add about ⅓ teaspoon of extra baking soda for each cup of juice.

When adding fruit juice to baked foods pat the fruit dry as extra moisture changes the batter and can cause under cooking in the center.

Non instant non fat milk has been processed less than instant and tends to retain more of the natural milk sweetness.

Fruit juice concentrates are available in the frozen foods case of most large grocery stores. Unsweetened juices are generally on the grocers shelves in bottles and cans. Health food stores carry the exotic and unusual juices which are fun to try and experiment with but tend to be a bit more costly than apple, orange, grape or pineapple.

STRAWBERRY SOUFFLE

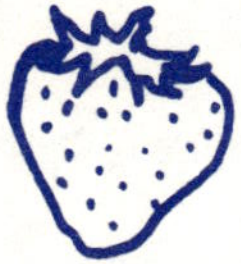

Serves 4
(Generously)
1 Serving Equals
1 Fruit Exchange
2 Fat Exchanges
130 Calories

C = 10 P = 0 F = 10

1 envelope unflavored gelatin
½ cup apple juice
2 teaspoons lemon juice
1 cup unsweetened pureed strawberries
(about 1-½ cups strawberries thawed (if frozen berries are used)
2 egg whites
1 cup whipped cream

In small sauce pan heat apple juice and gelatin until gelatin dissolves. Remove from heat and add pureed berries and lemon juice. Stir to mix well. Chill, stirring occasionally, until mixture mounds slightly when dropped from a spoon. Beat egg whites until stiff but not dry. Fold egg whites in gelatin mixture. Next fold whipped cream in berry/egg white mix. Turn into a 3 cup souffle dish with a 2 inch collar or a 4 cup dish without a collar. Refrigerate at least 4 hours before serving.

*May also be put in 4 individual souffle dishes.
*A real show stopper!

APPLESAUCE PANCAKES

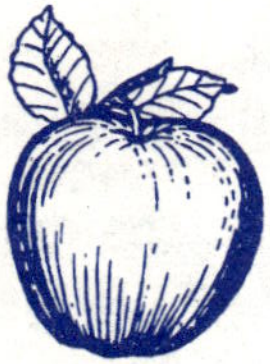

4 Servings
1 Serving = 125 Calories
1 Bread Exchange
1 Fat Exchange
¼ Fruit Exchange

C = 17.5 P = 2 F = 5

1 cup flour
¼ teaspoon salt
2 teaspoons baking powder
1 egg
1 cup milk
2 tablespoons oil
½ cup applesauce

Measure all ingredients and put in mixing bowl. Mix all ingredients until smooth. Cook on hot teflon griddle until bubbles form on one side. With a pancake turner carefully turn and brown on the other side.

These are special when topped with extra applesauce and sprinkled lightly with cinnamon.

QUICK ORANGE PANCAKES

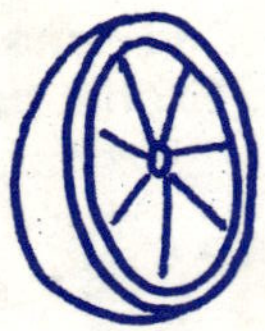

Serves 4
1 Serving Equals
1 Bread Exchange
1 Fat Exchange
¼ Milk Exchange
½ Fruit Exchange
155 Calories

C = 23 P = 4 F = 5

1 cup pancake mix
1 egg, beaten slightly
1 cup skim milk
¼ cup orange juice concentrate, thawed
½ teaspoon grated orange peel, if desired

Combine egg, milk and orange juice concentrate in small bowl. Stir in pancake flour and beat until most lumps disappear. Add orange peel, if desired. Cook on lightly greased or non-stick griddle until bubbles form. Turn with spatula and brown on other side. Serve warm.

Good with a fruit topping or syrup.

GERMAN PANCAKE

Serves 2
1 Serving Equals
¼ Milk Exchange
1-½ Bread Exchange
1 Medium Fat Meat Exchange
1-½ Fat Exchange
270 Calories

C = 24.5 P = 12 F = 13

½ cup skim milk
½ cup flour
2 eggs
1 tablespoon melted butter
little salt, cinnamon or nutmeg (3 shakes)

Beat together by hand first three ingredients. Melt butter in ovenproof frying pan. Pour all ingredients into frying pan. Sprinkle with spice. Bake at 425° for 12-15 minutes.

ENGLISH MUFFIN BREAD

Makes 16 slices
Each slice = 75 Calories
1 Bread Exchange
1 Milk Exchange (negligible)

C = 15 P = 2 F = 0

3 cups flour, divided
1 envelope (1 tablespoon) dry yeast
1 teaspoon salt
⅛ teaspoon baking soda
1 cup skim milk
¼ cup water
Corn meal (about 1 tablespoon)

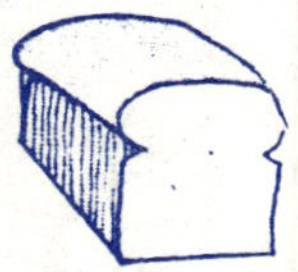

Combine 1-½ cups of the flour, the yeast, salt and baking soda in a large bowl. In a small saucepan, heat the milk and water until very warm (120 to 130 degrees). Add the liquids to the dry mixture and beat well. Stir in the remaining flour to make a stiff batter. Grease an 8-½ by 4-½ by 2-½ inch loaf pan; sprinkle with cornmeal. Place the batter in the pan and sprinkle the top lightly with cornmeal. Cover and let rise in a warm place for about 1 hour. Bake in 400-degree oven for 25 to 30 minutes, until done and lightly brown. Remove from the pan and cool upright on a baking rack.

Note: Batter bread of this type may also be baked in a glass or microwave-proof plastic loaf pan in a microwave oven. It should be baked for 6-½ minutes. It will not brown, but since this type of bread is usually toasted, anyway, the color is not as important as with some other breads.

*Great Toasted!

HOMEMADE RAISIN BREAD

Makes 2 loaves
= 32 slices
1 Slice = 70 Calories
1 Bread Exchange

C = 15 P = 2 F = 0

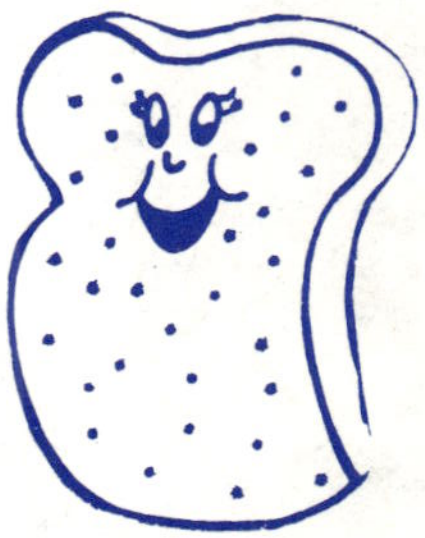

2 bread pans
4 cups unsifted flour
1 package active dry yeast
½ cup water
½ cup skim milk
½ cup butter or margarine (no shortening, please)
1 teaspoon salt
½ cup raisins
2 eggs
¼ cup chopped nuts

Mix 2 cups of the flour with the yeast in a large mixing bowl and set aside. In a medium saucepan mix water, milk, butter and salt and heat gently over low heat just until butter melts. Take off the burner and let cool for 5 minutes. Add the flour and yeast in large bowl. Mix well. Add the rest of the flour, raisins, eggs and nuts. Stir hard as dough will be stiff. Knead on a floured board (can be counter top or table) until dough is smooth and raisins are well mixed about. Divide the dough in half and shape into loaf. Place dough in bread pan that has been lightly greased

still more of the . . . **HOMEMADE RAISIN BREAD**

with shortening. Let rise in warm place (about 85°) *until nearly double in size. (Takes between an hour and an hour and a half). Bake at 375° about 35 minutes until top sounds hollow when tapped and cake tester comes out clean.*

°This is also fun to bake in 21-pound coffee cans. Just use the cans in place of the bread pans. It will rise to about 1 inch from the top when it's ready to bake. Fun for a party or picnics.

QUICK DONUTS

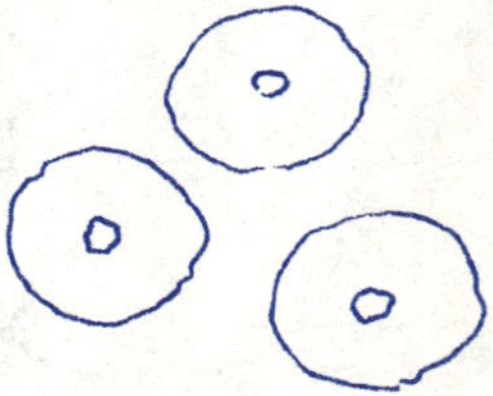

10 Servings
1 Serving = 95 Calories
1 Bread Exchange
½ Fat Exchange

C = 15 P = 2 F = 2.5

1 tube refrigerator biscuits
1 cup oil

Heat oil in small sauce pan with high sides. Flatten out biscuits and poke a hole in the middle with your finger. When oil begins to lightly smoke add biscuits one at a time. With tongs turn biscuits over when brown and fluffy. Remove and place on paper towel to cool. Super dipped in strawberry topping.

APPLE SWIRL BREAD

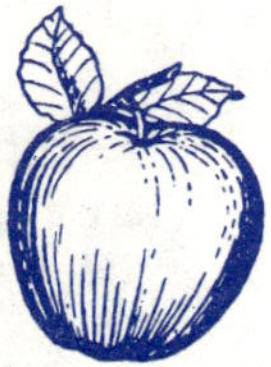

Makes 20 Slices
1 Bread Exchange
2/5 Fruit Exchange
⅓ Fat Exchange
97 Calories

C = 18.3 P = 2 F = 1.6

1 loaf frozen bread dough
2 tablespoons butter or margarine, room temperature
½ cup apple juice concentrate, room temperature
2 medium apples, peeled and chopped
½ teaspoon cinnamon

Let bread dough defrost until soft and pliable and starting to rise. With hands flatten into a rectangle about 8" x 14". Spread dough with butter or margarine – reserving 1 teaspoon to grease the bread pan. Mix chopped apples with 2-3 tablespoons apple juice concentrate and cinnamon. Put apple mixture on buttered dough. Roll dough jelly roll style from the 8" end. Pour remaining concentrate in buttered pan. Place roll in pan. Let rise until double in size. Preheat oven to 350°. Bake about 30 minutes, until brown and hollow sounding when tapped on top. Cool in pan 10 minutes. remove from pan carefully – syrup in bottom will be hot! Spoon syrup over top. Enjoy!

*This is always a diabetic class favorite!

RAISIN-APPLE STICKY BUNS

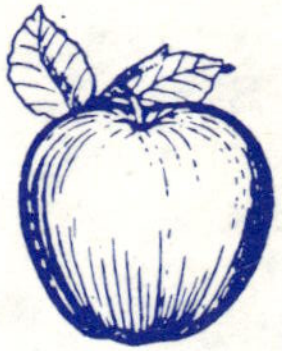

Makes 20 Rolls
1 Roll Equals (without nuts)
1 Bread Exchange
½ Fruit Exchange
⅓ Fat Exchange
105 Calories

C = 20 P = 2 F = 1.6

(with nuts) 1 Roll Equals
1 Bread Exchange
½ Fat Exchange
½ Fruit Exchange
113 Calories

C = 20 P = 2 F = 2.5

1 loaf frozen bread dough
2 tablespoons butter or margarine, room temperature
½ cup apple juice concentrate, room temperature
¼ cup raisins (golden are pretty)
2 medium apples, peeled and chopped
½ teaspoon cinnamon
¼ cup chopped walnuts – or pecans (if desired)

Remove dough from plastic package. Let dough defrost until soft, pliable and starting to rise. Divide in half. Flatten one half into rectangle about ⅓ inch thick. Spread with half of butter (reserve a bit of the butter – to lightly grease a 9 x 13 baking dish. Mix chopped apple, cinnamon, 2 tablespoons chopped nuts, raisins and 2 tablespoons apple juice concentrate. Pour remaining concentrate in lightly buttered pan. Sprinkle remaining nuts over apple juice concentrate in pan. Spread ½ apple filling mix over buttered rectangle. Roll jelly roll style from long side. Cut into 10 slices and place on nut/concentrate mix in pan. Repeat with remaining half of bread dough. Cover with clean towel and let rise until doubled. Preheat oven to 350°. Bake sticky buns 20-25 minutes until golden brown and hollow sounding when tapped. Let cool in pan 10 minutes. Invert on large serving platter and serve warm.

*May be baked in 2 - 8 inch round cake pans. *Best first day!

EASY DATE POCKETS

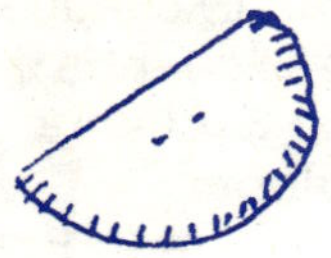

Makes 10
1 Serving Equals
1 Bread Exchange
⅓ Fruit Exchange
Fat Exchange negligible
85 Calories

C = 19 P = 2 F = 0

1 can buttermilk refrigerator* biscuits (the kind from the grocery store deli case)
10 teaspoons date spread (page 47)
1 teaspoon melted butter

Check can directions and preheat oven to specified temperature. Separate biscuits and flatten with palms of hands. Place 1 teaspoon date spread on one half of biscuit. Fold other half over filled side and press edges shut with tines of a fork. Brush with melted butter and bake on ungreased baking sheet according to directions on can.

EASY DATE NUT POCKETS

Makes 10
1 Bread Exchange
⅓ Fat Exchange
¼ Fruit Exchange
95 Calories
C = 19 P = 2 F = 1.25

Add two tablespoons chopped nuts to date filling. Follow directions for Easy Date Pockets.

EASY APPLE-RAISIN POCKETS

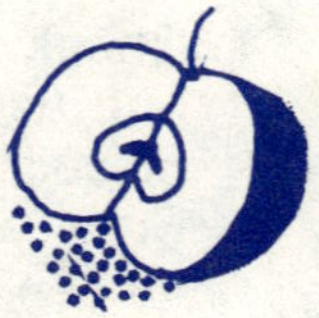

Makes 10
1 Serving Equals
1 Bread Exchange
⅓ Fruit Exchange
85 Calories

C = 19 P = 2 F = 0

Mix 1 chopped apple, two tablespoons raisins and a dash of cinnamon. Use one tablespoon filling per biscuit. Follow easy Date Pocket directions.

RAISIN-APPLESAUCE MUFFINS

1 large egg
2 tablespoons vegetable oil
1-½ cups unsweetened applesauce
2 cups flour
½ teaspoon baking soda
2 teaspoons baking powder
1 teaspoon cinnamon
¾ cup raisins
Preheat oven to 375°. Line muffin tin with muffin paper.

Makes 12
1 Muffin equals 1 Bread Exchange, ¾ Fruit Exchange
85 Calories
C = 30 P = 2 F = 0

Beat together egg, oil, and applesauce. Add flour, baking soda, baking powder, and cinnamon. Mix well. Stir in raisins. Spoon batter into muffin pans. Bake for 20 to 25 minutes or until firm to the touch and browned. Cool on wire racks. Serve warm.

RAISIN-NUT APPLESAUCE MUFFINS

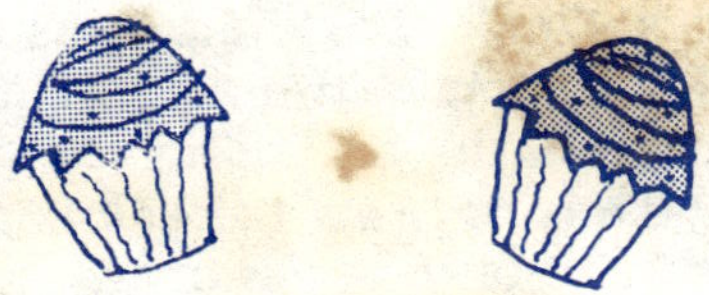

Makes 12
1 Muffin equals
1 Bread Exchange
¾ Fruit Exchange
⅓ Fat Exchange
100 calories
C = 30 P = 2 F = 2

Stir ¼ cup chopped walnuts to Raisin-Applesauce muffins when adding raisins.

ZUCCHINI BREAD

Serves 16
1 Slice Equals
½ Bread Exchange
1-½ Fat Exchange
½ Fruit Exchange
Vegetable negligible
Milk negligible
125 Calories

C = 13 P = 2 F = 7.5

½ cup zucchini, grated and patted dry
1-½ cups flour
¼ cup non fat dry milk powder
1 teaspoon baking soda
¼ teaspoon salt
⅓ cup oil
1 egg
1 8-¾ ounce can crushed pineapple in juice
½ cup raisins
½ cup chopped nuts

Preheat oven to 350°. Lightly grease a 9" x 5" x 3" loaf pan. Grate zucchini, squeeze out excess moisture and pat dry with paper toweling. Firmly pack ½ cup measuring cup. Mix together flour, dry milk powder, baking soda and salt. Set aside. In blender container puree pineapple with juice. Add oil and egg and blend. Add liquid ingredients to dry mixture. Mix well. Stir in zucchini, nuts and raisins. Pour batter into prepared pan. Bake 60-70 minutes – until nicely browned and cake tester comes out clean. Cool on wire rack before cutting.

*Sometimes I use half white – half whole wheat flour.
*If you object to raisins in zucchini bread – puree raisins with pineapple. They provide much sweetness to the zucchini bread.

ZUCCHINI GRIDDLE CAKES

Makes 8
1 Serving Equals 2 pancakes
½ Medium Fat Meat Exchange
1 Vegetable Exchange
¾ Bread Exchange
120 Calories

C = 17 P = 7 F = 2.5

4 cups grated zucchini
2 eggs, slightly beaten
½ cup bisquick

Preheat a griddle or electric fry pan to medium heat. Grease lightly. Combine all ingredients in a mixing bowl and thoroughly fold together. Scoop out zucchini mixture in a large serving spoon and form into patties on the griddle. Cook until brown on the bottom, then turn over with spatula. Cook until firm in the center and browned on the bottom.

*Good served with eggs in place of hash browns or any meat in place of potatoes.
*Really nice with fruit topping or spread – especially plum

CHEESY ZUCCHINI GRIDDLE CAKES

Makes 8
1 Serving Equals 2 pancakes
½ Medium Fat Meat Exchange
¼ High Fat Meat Exchange
1 Vegetable Exchange
¾ Bread Exchange
145 Calories

C = 17 P = 9 F = 4.5

These are original recipes shared by marathon runner Steve Timm.

Add ¼ cup grated sharp cheddar and 1 tablespoon chopped pimiento if desired to Zucchini Griddle Cakes above. Dust with 1 sweep of fresh ground black pepper.

SWEET FRUIT SOUP

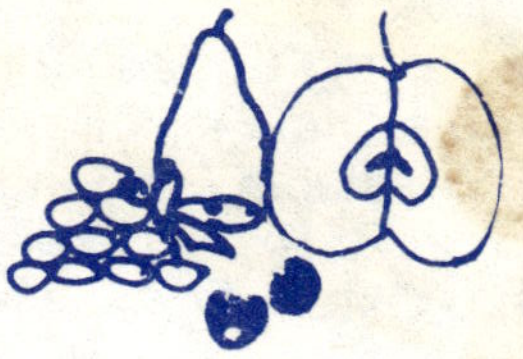

Serves 8
1 Serving Equals
1-½ Fruit Exchange
60 Calories

C = 15 P = 0 F = 0

1 8 ounce package mixed dried fruit (apples, pears, prunes, apricots w/o pits)
½ cup light or golden raisins
1-½ cups water
¼ cup tapioca
1 cup red or light grape juice
1 stick cinnamon

In sauce pan combine tapioca and water over medium heat and bring to boil. Cut the dried fruit in bite size pieces. Add raisins, dried fruit pieces and cinnamon stick. Simmer until fruit is tender and thickened (30-40 minutes). Stir in grape juice. Remove cinnamon stick and enjoy!

Good hot or cold. Refrigerate any leftovers.

*Great first course at brunch – festive served in a stemmed glass.
*Nice for dessert with a dollop of whipped cream.
*Thickens a bit when left over and may be enjoyed heated and used as a topping for waffles or pancakes.

SPICY MANDARIN ORANGES

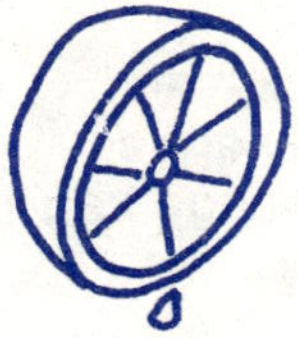

Serves 6
1 Serving Equals
1 Fruit Exchange
40 Calories
C = 10 P = 0 F = 0
With 1 tablespoon whipped cream, add ½ fat exchange
23 calories
2.5 gm fat

1 11 ounce can unsweetened mandarin oranges in fruit juice
1-½ cups orange juice
4 teaspoons minute tapioca
¼ teaspoon ground ginger or cinnamon

Drain juice from mandarin oranges and mix with orange juice and tapioca in sauce pan. Over low heat, cook stirring occasionally until mixture boils. Remove from heat and stir in spice. Add drained oranges stirring gently to mix but not breaking fruit sections. Cool. Serve lukewarm or chilled.

*Excellent topped with a dollop of whipped cream.

*A brunch treat served warm on a waffle and sprinkled with a pinch of shredded coconut.

*Served cold in individual dishes for dessert with whipped cream it's fruit pudding.

APRICOT WHIP

Serves 4
1 Serving Equals
1 Fruit Exchange
Meat Exchange negligible
40 Calories
a
C = 10 P = 0 F = 0

16 apricot halves canned in juice or water
1 envelope unflavored gelatin
¼ teaspoon almond extract
¼ cup boiling water
2 egg whites

Place apricot halves in blender container and blend until smooth. Dissolve gelatin in boiling water and stir into apricot mix with almond extract. Refrigerate until slightly thickened. Beat egg whites until stiff (but not dry) and fold into apricot mix. Spoon into serving dishes and refrigerate.

*Pretty served in a stemmed (wine type) glass garnished with a fresh fruit bit or lemon twist.

BAKED PEAR ON THE HALF SHELL

Serves 4
1 Serving Equals
1-½ Fruit Exchange

2 fresh baking pears (Bosc are best)
3 tablespoons apple pear concentrate
5 tablespoons boiling water
½ teaspoon cinnamon
Raisin or date filling (below)

Raising Filling
Combine ¼ cup raisins and 2 tablespoons chopped walnuts.

Date Filling
Combine 4 chopped dates, 2 tablespoons chopped nuts and ½ teaspoon grated orange peel (optional).

Preheat oven to 350°. Halve and core pear. Fill each center with one fourth of the raisin or date filling and place in a 8 inch square baking dish. Combine boiling water, concentrate and cinnamon and pour over pears. Bake 35-40 minutes, until tender, basting frequently with syrup.

*Good warm or cold.

BAKED APPLES ON THE HALF SHELL

Substitute apples for pears and apple juice concentrate for apple pear concentrate. Values are the same as if using pears.

APPLESAUCE

Serves 6
1 Serving Equals
1 Fruit Exchange
40 Calories

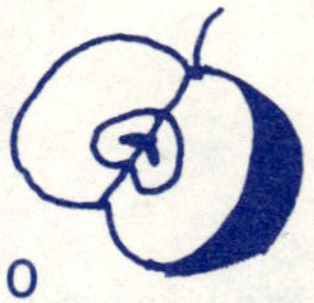

4 medium peeled, sliced apples
¼ cup apple juice concentrate
½ cup water
cinnamon or nutmeg to taste

C = 10 P = 0 F = 0

Combine all ingredients in saucepan. Simmer covered until apples are tender – about 15-20 minutes. Stir to mix well and break up slices. May seive if desired. Delicious warm or cold. *If apples are very juicy, you may want to add only ¼ cup water.

*Quick trick – If you're in a hurry unpeeled apples may be used. Simply cook until tender and strain or seive apples. Sauce will be fine textured. Season after straining.
*Apple juice may be substituted for the concentrate and water, however, you do not have the control of liquid concentrate in the sweetener.

RAISIN BAKED APPLES

Serves 4
1 Serving Equals
2 Fruit Exchanges
80 Calories

4 medium apples
¼ cup raisins
⅔ cup apple juice
cinnamon, nutmeg or apple pie spice (optional)

C = 20 P = 0 F = 0

Preheat oven to 375°. Wash and core apples. Peel a collar off the top of each apple and if apple won't sit up take a small slice from the bottom. Place in baking dish. Fill each apple center with one tablespoon raisins. Pour juice over apples and sprinkle lightly with spice, if desired. Bake 40-45 minutes until firm, soft, basting frequently. Serve warm or chilled.

Super dessert with a dollop of whipped cream.

INDIVIDUAL APPLESAUCE SOUFFLE

2 cups unsweetened applesauce
2 tablespoons frozen apple juice concentrate
1 teaspoon grated orange peel, if desired
¼ teaspoon cinnamon or nutmeg
4 egg whites

Serves 6
1 Serving = Equals
1 Fruit Exchange
40 Calories

C = 10 P = 0 F = 0

In a small bowl mix applesauce, apple juice concentrate, orange peel, and spice. Set aside. Beat egg whites until stiff and glossy. Fold applesauce mix into egg whites gently. Spoon immediately into custard cups or individual ramkins. Bake at 350° until lightly browned – 15 to 20 minutes. Serve immediately – warm.

*This recipe is easily cut in half to make only 3 servings.

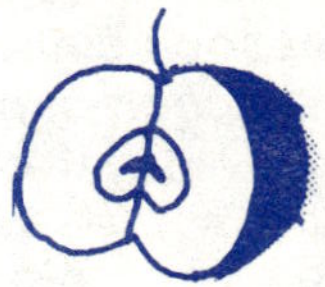

BAKED APPLES

4 medium apples
⅔ cup apple juice
½ teaspoon cinnamon or apple pie spice

Serves 4
1 Serving Equals
1-½ Fruit Exchanges
60 Calories

C = 15 P = 0 F = 0

Preheat oven to 375°. Wash and core apples. Peel a collar off the top of each apple (if apple won't sit up – take a small slice from the bottom). Place in baking dish. Mix apple juice and spice. Pour over apples. Bake 40-45 minutes until firm, soft, basting frequently. Serve warm or chilled spooning syrup over apples.

"ADULT" BAKED PEARS

Serves 8
1 Serving =
1 Fruit Exchange
* alcohol evaporates from wine
40 Calories

C = 10 P = 0 F = 0

4 fresh pears
1 cup red grape juice
½ cup dry white wine
½ teaspoon cinnamon
1 tablespoon cornstarch
½ cup cold water

Halve and core pears and place cut side up in baking dish. (If skins are tender they may be left on – otherwise peal pears) Mix grape juice, wine and cinnamon. Pour over pears. Cover and bake at 350° until tender – about 30 minutes. Mix cornstarch and water in small sauce pan. Add liquid from pear and cook until thickened. Pour sauce over pears. Good warm or cold.

APPLES 'n APRICOTS

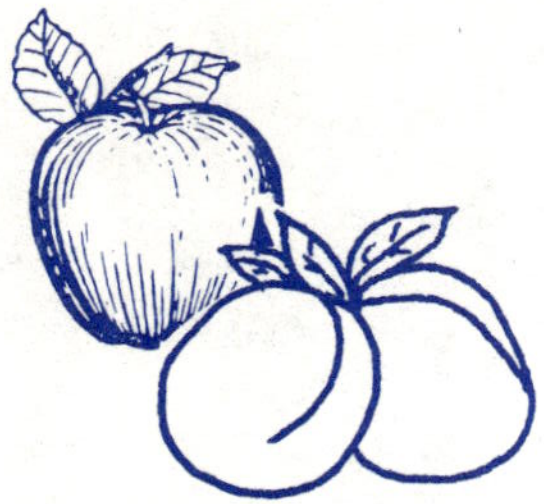

Serves 2
1 Serving Equals
2 Fruit Exchange
80 Calories

C = 20 P = 0 F = 0

AS A TOPPING
Serves 4
1 Serving Equals
1 Fruit Exchange

C = 10 P = 0 F = 0

8 apricot halves, canned in juice or water
1 small apple, cored and diced
½ cup orange juice
1 cinnamon stick
2-3 whole cloves

Drain apricots and combine with diced apple (peel adds color but may be removed if you prefer), orange juice, cinnamon stick and cloves in small sauce pan. Cook over medium heat 2-3 minutes (if you like a bit of crunch) or simmer 8-10 minutes for soft fruit. Remove cinnamon stick and cloves and enjoy!

*Great breakfast fruit on a cold morning!
*Good topping for waffles, french toast or pancakes.
*Serve leftovers cold for dessert!

PEAR CLOWNS

Makes 2
1 Serving Equals
½ Fruit Exchange
Vegetable negligible
20 Calories

C = 5 P = 0 F = 0

What child can resist a dessert that smiles?

1 peeled fresh or canned pear, halved
4 raisins
1 fresh carrot-grated or in curls
1 cherry, sliced

Place pear cut side down on small plate. Use raisins for eyes and cherry pieces for nose and mouth. Garnish with carrot hair. A real treat for little ones.

GRANNY PEARS

1 peeled fresh or canned pear, halved
½ cup cottage cheese
4 raisins
1 cherry, sliced
2 lettuce leaves (curly is best – red or green)

Follow directions for Pear Clowns except place pear half on lettuce leaf for bonnet and make cottage cheese hair. Add 1 medium fat meat exchange, 75 calories and 7 grams protein, 5 grams fat to Pear Clowns.

PINEAPPLE ICE

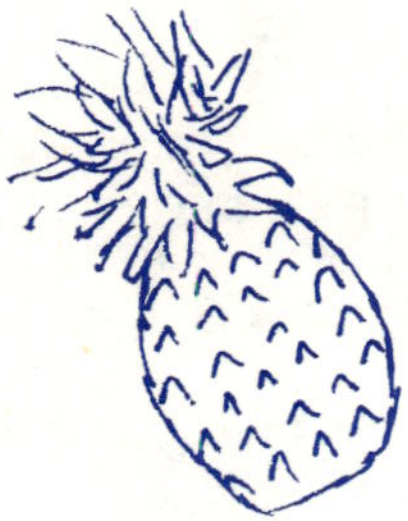

Makes 1 Quart
Serves 6
1 Serving Equals
1 Fruit Exchange
45 Calories

C = 11 P = 0 F = 0

1-½ teaspoons unflavored gelatin (½ envelope)
1 cup pineapple juice (canned – fresh will not set up)
1 tablespoon lemon juice
1 cup canned crushed pineapple in juice undrained
1 egg white, stiffly beaten

Mix gelatin, pineapple juice, lemon juice and pineapple in sauce pan. Bring to a full boil. Remove from heat and allow to cool. Pour into freezer tray (ice cube tray with grid network works well) and allow to freeze until mushy. Remove from freezer and beat until fluffy. Fold in beaten egg white. Freeze until firm, stirring twice.

STRAWBERRY-PINEAPPLE OR RASPBERRY-PINEAPPLE ICE

May substitute 1 cup crushed strawberries or raspberries for cup of crushed pineapple for an interesting change.

FRUIT CUP

½ Cup = 40 Calories
1 Fruit Exchange

C = 10 P = 0 F = 0

Fresh fruit is colorful, tasty and refreshing, and a mixture in a bright dish is welcomed by everyone!

One-half cup of any combination of the following equals 1 fruit exchange.

Apples, oranges, berries, grapefruit, nectarines, peaches, pears, pineapple or tangerines.

*To serve I usually cut the oranges in half and save the peel for fruit cups.

For a large group it's fun to put all the fruit in a pineapple shell for the serving bowl. Aloha!

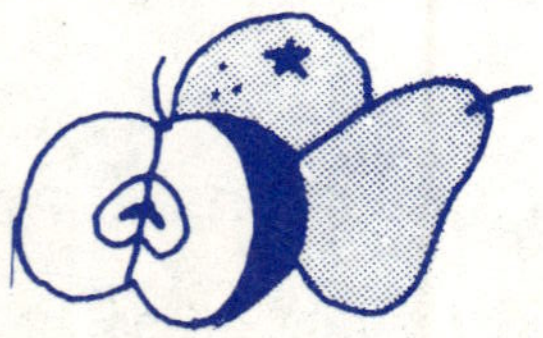

FRUIT GEL

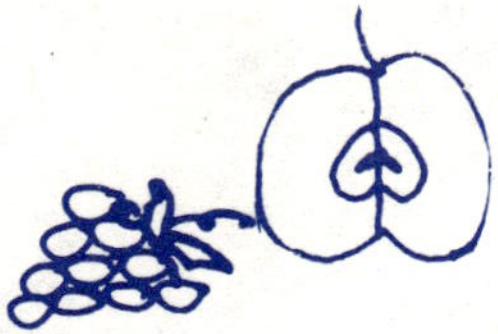

Grape Gel serves 8
Apple Gel serves 6
Orange gel serves 4

1 Fruit Exchange =
40 Calories

C = 10 P = 0 F = 0

Make your own gelatin by heating one cup of fruit juice and one envelope unflavored gelatin. When mixture boils add one cup of cold juice. This has super flavor and servings are equal to the amount of juice allowed for the fruit exchange of the type of juice used. Grape and apple are my favorites.

For dessert top with whipped cream.

FRUITY WHIP

1 Fruit Exchange
40 Calories

C = 10 P = 0 F = 0

Prepare fruit gel in a large mixing bowl. Chill stirring occasionally until almost set. (Will be very thick and get lumpy when stirred.) Remove from refrigerator and beat at high speed with mixer until foamy and about triple in volume. Pour into a large mold or individual serving dishes and chill until set.

JELLED FRUIT WHIP PARFAITS

1 Fruit Exchange =
40 Calories

C = 10 P = 0 F = 0

Make basic fruit gel. Pour half mixture into stem type dessert or parfait glasses. Refrigerate individual glasses and remaining gelatin/juice mix. When remaining gelatin/juice mix gets syrupy beat with mixer to foam. Spoon foam in equal amounts on gelatin in individual dishes. Refrigerate until firm.

*Nice cool light dessert.
*Really extends fruit exchanges!

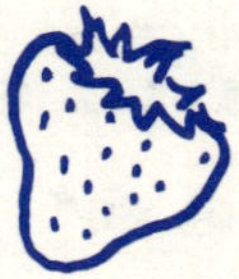

FRUIT GELATIN DESSERT

Serves 4
1 Serving Equals
1-¼ Fruit Exchange
½ Fat Exchange
75 Calories

C = 50 P = 0 F = 2.5

1 cup red grape juice
1 cup boiling water
1 envelope unflavored gelatin
¾ cup sliced strawberries
¼ cup (4 tablespoons) whipped cream

Combine gelatin and juice in small bowl stirring to dissolve gelatin. Add boiling water and stir to mix. Divide berries equally into four dessert dishes. Pour gelatin mix over top. Chill until set. Top with whipped cream – 1 tablespoon per serving.

FRUITY DESSERT TOPPING

Makes 1-½ cups
Serves 8
1 Serving Equals
1 Fat Exchange
⅛ Fruit Exchange
50 Calories

½ cups whipping cream (1 cup whipped)
½ cup canned crushed pineapple in juice

C = 1.25 P = 0 F = 5

Drain pineapple while whipping cream. Blot drained pineapple on paper towels. Fold pineapple in whipped cream. Cover and chill.

*Too much pineapple juice will cause the topping to be runny.
*Delicious on fresh, or frozen or canned fruit.
*For an elegant touch anytime place fruit in a stemmed glass and top with fruity dessert topping!

FRUIT PARFAIT

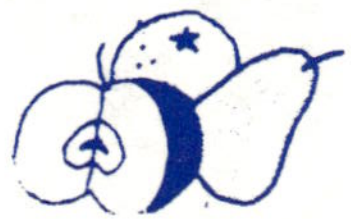

Serves 1
1 Serving Equals
1-⅛ Fruit Exchange
1 Fat Exchange
90 Calories

C = 11.25 P = 0 F = 5

3 tablespoons fruity dessert topping
½ cup peaches, pears, raspberries, blueberries, chopped orange or pineapple chunks

Wash and drain fruit, if fresh, dicing peaches, pears. (Drain if using juice packed, canned fruit) Place one tablespoon fruity dessert topping in bottom of parfait glass. Layer with ¼ cup fruit, another tablespoon topping, remaining ¼ cup fruit and remaining topping.

SUNSHINE GELATIN

My daughter Carrie's favorite

Serves 6
1 Serving Equals
1 Fruit Exchange
⅓ Vegetable Exchange
49 Calories
C = 12 P = .5 F = 0

¾ cup orange juice
1 8-¾ ounce can crushed pineapple in pineapple juice
1 envelope unflavored gelatin
1 cup grated carrot

Place gelatin in ¼ cup orange juice to soften. Bring remaining orange juice to a boil. Mix in juice/gelatin and stir until dissolved. Add pineapple with juice and grated carrot. Stir well. Pour into mold and refrigerate until firm.

SCOTT'S WATERMELON

"Fun summertime gelatin"

Without raisins serves 5
With raisins serves 6
1 Serving Equals
1 Fruit Exchange
40 Calories

C = 10 P = 0 F = 0

2-½ cups watermelon chunks, seeds & rind removed
1 cup mashed strawberries
2 envelopes unflavored gelatin
⅓ cup apple or orange juice
2 tablespoons raisins (optional)

Without Raisins:
Mix gelatin and fruit juice and set aside to soften. Place watermelon chunks and strawberries in blender and puree. Add juice/gelatin and mix well. Pour into mold and refrigerate until firm.

With Raisins:
Remove watermelon flesh and seeds carefully from a small watermelon reserving ½ the "shell" for a mold. Follow directions above except stir raisins in mix before pouring into watermelon rind. Refrigerate until firm and serve in slices. This is super fun for a picnic . . . a seedless non-drip watermelon! (Recipe may be doubled to fill watermelon shell.
*A summer watermelon dessert was a special request of Portland KXL radio personality Scott Carter, an advocate of things good and sugar-free.

APPLE SYRUP

Makes 1-¾ cups
9 Servings
1 Serving Equals
1 Fruit Exchange

C = 10 P = 0 F = 0

1 6 ounce can frozen apple juice concentrate, unsweetened
1 tablespoon cornstarch
1 cup cold water
¼ teaspoon cinnamon, nutmeg or apple pie spice

Mix cornstarch in ½ cup water until smooth. Combine cornstarch mix, remaining water and concentrate in saucepan. Cook over medium heat, stirring constantly, until syrup thickens. Season with spice to taste. Serve warm. Refrigerate leftovers – reheat before serving. Will keep up to 10 days.

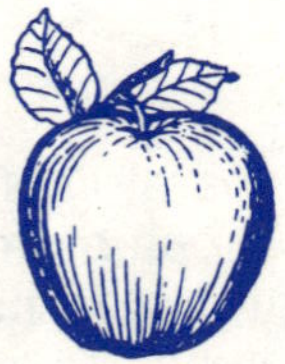

SAUCY PINEAPPLE SYRUP

Serves 8
1 Serving Equals
½ Fruit Exchange
20 Calories

C = 5 P = 0 F = 0

1 8 ounce can crushed pineapple in unsweetened juice
½ - ¾ teaspoon tapioca or cornstarch
¼ cup cold water
dash of cinnamon, if desired

Mix thickener in water. Combine all ingredients except cinnamon, in saucepan. Cook over medium-low heat until mixture thickens. Season with cinnamon if desired.

*Super on waffles – for a festive south of the border touch – sprinkle with unsweetened coconut.
*Tapioca makes the sauce a bit thicker and adds texture.
*For a smooth syrup, puree all ingredients in blender until smooth, transfer to saucepan and cook until thickened.

APPLE-CRANBERRY SAUCE

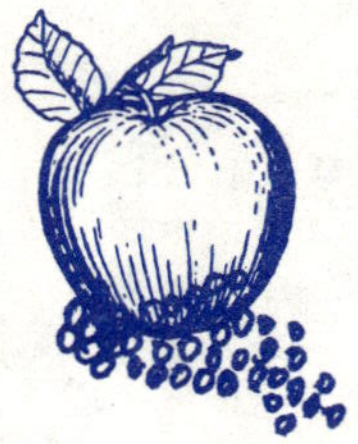

Serves 8
1 Serving Equals
1 Fruit Exchange
40 Calories

C = 10 P = 0 F = 0

1 cup cranberries
¼ cup apple juice concentrate
1-½ cup apple juice
1 tablespoon orange juice concentrate
2 tablespoons cornstarch

Wash berries and pick out any that are brown. Mix apple juice concentrate, apple juice, orange juice concentrate and cornstarch in saucepan stirring to mix and dissolve cornstarch. Stir in cranberries. Cook over medium heat until cranberries pop. Serve warm or cold.

*These are good with a cinnamon stick cooked in the sauce for a spicy flavor.
*Cranberries freeze well. In the fall buy several bags and freeze in bags until time to cook.

PLUM CONSERVE

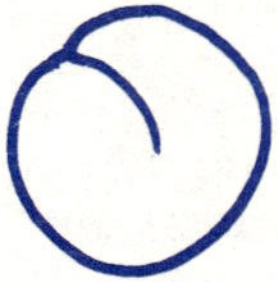

Makes 1-½ Cups
1 Tablespoon Equals
¾ Fruit Exchange
1/5 Fat Exchange
39 Calories
C = 7.5 P = 0 F = 1

1 cup soft pitted prunes
½ cup apple juice concentrate
½ teaspoon cinnamon
¼ cup chopped walnuts

Place concentrate in blender on low speed to slush if not defrosted. Add prunes and blend until thick and creamy. Pour into "jam jar" and stir in chopped nuts.

*Super on hot toast or rolls.

PRUNE SPREAD

Makes 1-¼ Cups
1 Tablespoon Equals
¾ Fruit Exchange
30 Calories

C = 7.5 P = 0 F = 0

1 cup soft pitted prunes
½ cup apple juice concentrate
½ teaspoon cinnamon

Place concentrate in blender on low speed to slush if not defrosted. Add prunes and blend until thick and creamy. Refrigerate until needed.

*Great with peanut butter!

QUICK PEACH BUTTER

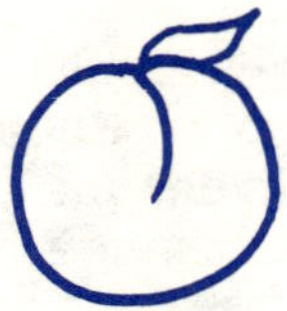

Makes 2-½ cups
2 Tablespoons Equals
¼ Fruit Exchange
10 Calories

C = 2.5 P = 0 F = 0

1 16 ounce can juice packed peaches, sliced
1 envelope unflavored gelatin
½ cup unsweetened apple juice
¼ teaspoon cinnamon or apple pie spice

Drain peach juice into blender container. Add gelatin and let set 2 minutes to soften. Bring apple juice to boil while gelatin softens and add to container. Blend on high until dissolved. Add fruit & spice and blend until smooth. Taste and adjust spice. Refrigerate until set.

*Take out of refrigerator when beginning meal preparation and allow to come to room temperature to enhance flavor
*Good spread for biscuits and toast.
*Yummy with peanut butter.

QUICK APRICOT BUTTER: Substitute juice packed apricots for peaches. Values are the same as with peaches.

DATE BUTTER

Makes 1 cup
1 Tablespoon Equals
1 Fruit Exchange
40 Calories

$C = 10$ $P = 0$ $F = 0$

1 cup chopped dates (not sugared)
½ cup water

Place dates and water in covered saucepan. Cook covered over very low heat until dates become very soft. Pour into blender and blend until thick and smooth. Store in refrigerator.

DATE-NUT BUTTER

Makes 1 cup
1 Tablespoon Equals
1 Fruit Exchange
¼ Fat Exchange
51 Calories

$C = 10$ $P = 0$ $F = 25$

Make date butter stirring in ¼ cup chopped walnuts after blending.

*If packaged chopped dates are unavailable without sugar – simply buy whole dates and chop. Remove pits before cooking if they are still in the whole date.
*Date butter and Date-Nut Butter are excellent fillings for cookies and breakfast rolls.
*Excellent sandwich filling for dark or nut breads mixed with cream cheese.

FRUIT BUTTER

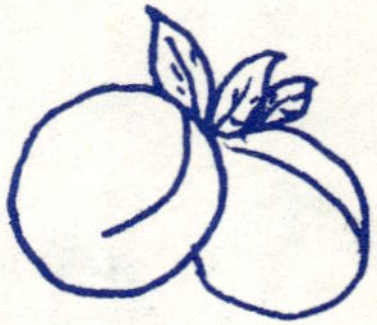

1 Tablespoon Equals
20 Calories
½ Fruit Exchange

C = 5 P = 0 F = 0

10 dried apricots
½ cup raisins
2 medium apples, peeled and sliced
½ teaspoon cinnamon

Place apples in blender and blend about 30 seconds to form some liquid, add raisins and apricots and blend until thick and smooth. Store in refrigerator.

Good on warm biscuits, toast or bagels with cream cheese.

EASY STRAWBERRY JAM

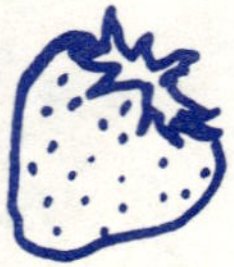

Makes Approx. 2-½ cups
1 Tablespoon Equals
¼ Fruit Exchange
10 Calories

C = 2.5 P = 0 F = 0

1 envelope unflavored gelatin
4 teaspoons tapioca
½ cup unsweetened white grape juice (undiluted)
2 teaspoon fresh lemon juice
2 cups mashed-fully ripe strawberries

Wash and mash berries. Combine the gelatin, tapioca, grape juice and lemon juice in sauce pan. Stir and let stand 2 minutes. Over medium heat, stirring constantly dissolve gelatin. (Takes about 2 minutes). Add the berries and bring to a boil, stirring constantly. Reduce heat and simmer uncovered about 5 minutes. Cool and refrigerate.

FRENCH PASTRY ICING

Makes 1 Cup
1 Serving Equals
2 Tablespoons
3 Fat Exchanges
¾ Fruit Exchange
170 Calories

1 cube butter or margarine, room temperature
½ cup apple juice concentrate, defrosted
4-½ teaspoons flour
cinnamon or nutmeg to taste

C = 8 P = 0 F = 15

With wire whip blend apple juice concentrate and flour in small saucepan. Cook over medium heat until thick and glossy. Remove from heat and allow to cool completely. In a small mixing bowl beat butter to light and fluffy. Add thickened concentrate in 3 additions beating well. Season to taste. Spread on your favorite goodie.

*This icing may be thickened slightly and can be colored for a decorator icing.
*Orange and pineapple juice concentrates may be substituted for the apple for a flavor change. *Very rich and sweet.

CAROB GLAZE

1 tablespoon butter or margarine, room temperature
½ cup carob powder
7 tablespoons water
1 teaspoon vanilla

Makes about ¾ cup

1 teaspoon – negligible

Combine all ingredients in saucepan over medium heat. Cook, stirring occasionally until glaze thickens. Drizzle as desired. If glaze thickens too much before it is all used, just reheat slightly to return to "drizzle" consistency.

MERINGUE

Serves 8
Exchanges Negligible
5 Calories

3 egg whites
¼ teaspoon cream of tartar
4 teaspoons apple juice concentrate, thawed

C = 1.25 P = 0 F = 0

Beat egg whites until frothy. Add cream of tartar and beat until stiff peaks form, but not dry. Add concentrate and continue beating until well blended. Top desired dish and bake in preheated 425° oven about 5 minutes until curls are lightly browned and. set.

*Make curls and swirls with back of spoon.

ORANGE TOPPING

Makes 1 Cup
2 Tablespoons Equals
⅛ Milk Exchange
15 Calories
Fruit Exchange negligible

⅓ cup non fat dry milk powder
⅓ cup ice cold orange juice

C = 2 P = 1 F = 0

Mix milk powder and orange juice in small mixing bowl. Beat on high until stiff. Store covered in refrigerator.

*Kids enjoy their fruit cups (fresh fruit served in half orange shells) frosted with orange topping and decorated with raisin faces!
*Great on fruit salad.

SUGARFREE APPLE PIE

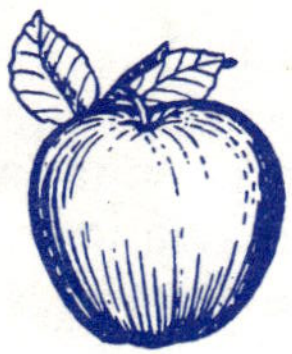

Makes 8 Servings
1 Serving (including the crust) =
220 Calories
1-½ Fruit Exchanges
1 Bread Exchange
2 Fat Exchanges

C = 30 P = 2 F = 10

4 cups sliced peeled apples (sweet varieties are best)
½ cup frozen apple juice concentrate, undiluted
1-½ to 2 teaspoons tapioca, cornstarch or flour (see note)
½ teaspoon lemon juice, optional
½ to 1 teaspoon cinnamon, nutmeg or apple pie spice

Divide pastry into 2 parts and roll thin to fit an 8 or 9 inch plate. Set aside.

Mix apples, apple juice concentrate, thickener and spice and stir until apples are well-coated. Add lemon juice, if desired, to keep apples lighter-colored. Taste 1 piece of apple to check the spice. Pour into the pastry-lined pie pan and top with the second crust or pastry strips. Seal the edges and cut slits in the top crust to allow steam to escape. Bake at 425 degrees for 40-45 minutes, until golden brown. Serve warm or cold.

Note: Apples have some natural pectin, but a small amount of thickener seems necessary to "hold" the sweet concentrate of the apples for an even flavor.

DEEP DISH APPLE PIE

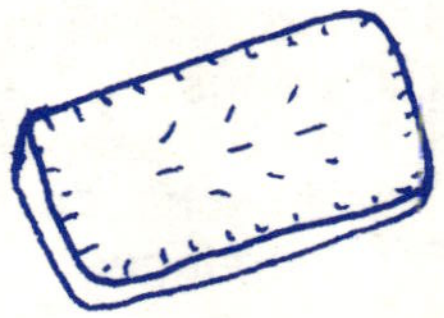

Serves 16
1 Serving Equals
1-½ Fruit Exchange
½ Bread Exchange
1 Fat Exchange
140 Calories

C = 23 P = 1 F = 5

Make sugar free apple pie – doubling the amount of the filling. Place in 9 x 13 baking dish. Roll out the pastry crust for 2 crust 8" pie into rectangle to top baking dish with crust sealing edges. Cut slits in top and bake at 425° about 45 minutes until golden brown and bubbly.

Only has one crust – same great taste – fewer calories. Great for large groups. Generous servings.

*This pie is a real favorite and enjoyed by everyone!
*Great with a slice of cheddar cheese.

PEACH PIE

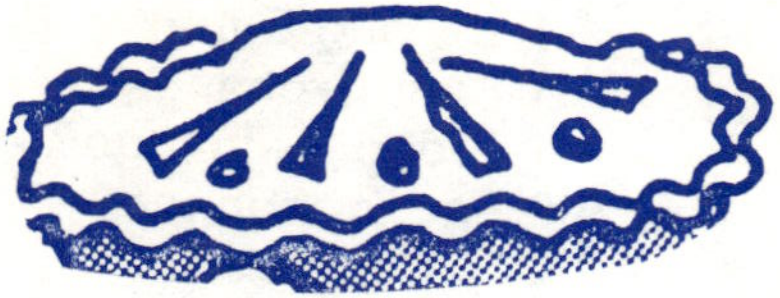

Serves 8
1 Serving Equals
1 Fruit Exchange
1 Bread Exchange
2 Fat Exchanges
200 Calories
C = 25 P = 2 F = 10

Pastry Crust for 8" 2 crust pie (page 63)
1 16 ounce can sliced peaches canned in fruit juice undrained
2 tablespoons quick cooking tapioca
2 drops almond extract
½ teaspoon cinnamon

Divide pastry into 2 parts and roll them to fit an 8 inch pie plate. Line bottom of pie plate and set aside.

Preheat oven to 425°. Mix peaches and juice, tapioca, almond extract and cinnamon. Pour into prepared unbaked pie crust and top with second crust. Seal the edges and cut slits in top to allow steam to escape. Bake for 40-45 minutes in preheated oven – until golden brown. Serve warm or cold.

EARLY AMERICAN PEAR PIE

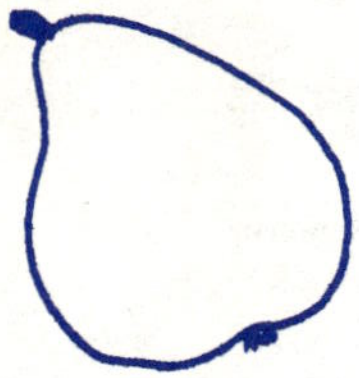

Serves 8
1 Serving Equals
1 Fruit Exchange
1 Bread Exchange
2 Fat Exchanges
200 Calories
C = 25 P = 2 F = 10

Pastry crust for 8" 2 crust pie
1 16 ounce can pears canned in fruit juice, undrained
2 tablespoons quick cooking tapioca
¾ teaspoon cinnamon or nutmeg

Divide pastry into 2 parts and roll thin to fit an 8 inch pie plate. Line bottom of pie plate and set aside.

Preheat oven to 425°. Slice pear halves. Mix pears and juice, tapioca and spice. Pour into prepared unbaked pie shell and top with second crust. Seal the edges and cut slits in the top to allow the steam to escape. Bake for 40-45 minutes in preheated oven until golden brown. Serve warm or cold.

RAISIN PIE

Serves 8
1 Serving Equals
1 Bread Exchange
2 Fat Exchanges
1-½ Fruit Exchanges
220 Calories

C = 30 P = 2 F = 10

*with nuts add 1 fat exchange,
45 calories and 5 grams fat

Pastry crust for 8 inch pie (page 63)
1-½ cups seedless raisins
½ cup boiling apple juice
1 cup boiling water
1-½ tablespoons flour or cornstarch
1-½ teaspoons grated lemon rind
2 tablespoons lemon juice
½ cup nuts (optional)*

Make pastry for 2 crust pie. Line bottom of 8" pie plate with half crust. Set aside. Prehat oven to 425°. In small saucepan cook raisins in water and apple juice (about 5 minutes) until tender. Stir in flour or cornstarch and stir constantly (about 2 minutes) until thickened. Remove from heat and add remaining ingredients. Pour hot filling into unbaked pastry shell. Top with remaining crust. Seal edges and cut vents to allow steam to escape. Bake 30-40 minutes – until golden brown.

*A Thanksgiving classic.

FROZEN STRAWBERRY PIE

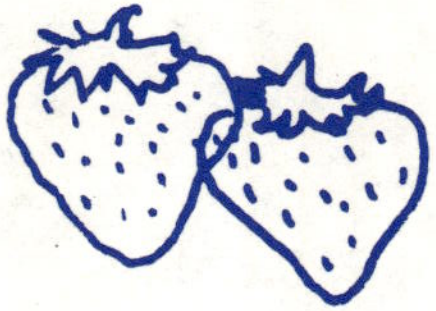

Serves 8
1 Serving Equals
2-¾ Fat Exchanges
¾ Bread Exchange
½ Fruit Exchange
½ Medium Fat Meat Exchange
250 Calories

C = 17 P = 5 F = 18.75

1 graham cracker crust (page 64)
1 8 ounce package neufchatel cheese, room temperature
1 cup sour cream (not imitation)
2 10 ounce packages non sugared frozen strawberries, defrosted

Blend cheese and sour cream. Reserve ½ cup berries and set aside. Mix remaining berries and any juice in cheese/sour cream base. Pour into crust and freeze until firm. Remove from freezer 5 minutes before serving. Cut into wedges and spoon 1 tablespoon reserved berries and juice over each wedge.

*Great hot weather dessert – cool and slightly tangy.

FROZEN BLUEBERRY PIE

Substitute frozen blueberries for strawberries.

STRAWBERRY CHIFFON PIE

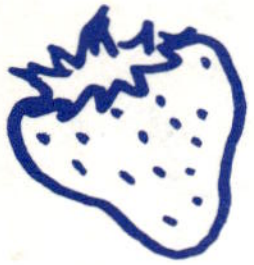

Serves 8
1 Serving Equals
2 Fat Exchanges
½ Bread Exchange
¾ Fruit Exchange
155 Calories

C = 15 P = 1 F = 10

1 8 inch baked pastry shell (1 crust type)
1 pint fully ripe fresh strawberries
1 envelope unflavored gelatin
¾ cup apple or apple-pear juice
1 teaspoon lemon juice
2 egg whites
1 cup whipped cream

Crush strawberries and add ¼ cup apple or apple-pear juice. Soften gelatin in remaining ½ cup juice and dissolve over low heat. Allow juice/gelatin to cool slightly and mix with berries and lemon juice. Chill, stirring occasionally until partially set. (It's important that the gelatin be just the right consistency – partially set but still pourable. Beat egg whites to form soft peaks. Fold in strawberry mixture, then whipped cream. Chill until strawberry filling mounds but is not firm. Pile high into cooled pie shell and chill until firm.

Pretty trimmed with whipped cream stars and fresh berry halves. For special occasions trim with berry halves and silver leaves.

FRENCH BERRY GLAZE PIE

Serves 8
1 Serving Equals
½ Bread Exchange
1-½ Fat Exchanges
½ Medium Fat Meat Exchange
1 Fruit Exchange
180 Calories

C = 17.5 P = 4.5 F = 10

1 baked 9" pie shell, cooled
1 quart fresh sliced strawberries, raspberries, blackberries or blueberries
1 cup apple juice
2-½-3 tablespoons cornstarch
1 8 ounce package Neufchatel cheese, room temperature

Wash and drain berries, slicing strawberries only. Simmer 1 cup berries in ⅔ cup apple juice 3 minutes. Blend in cornstarch and stir constantly 1 minute over medium high heat – until mixture thickens. Remove from heat and cool. Spread softened cheese in baked shell. Top with 2-½ cups berries (save ½ cup to garnish). Cover with cooked fruit mixture and garnish with berries. Refrigerate 2-3 hours until firm. Enjoy!

*Luscious and rich with a dollop of whipped cream.

JELLED BERRY PIE

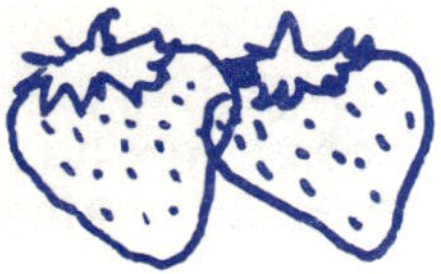

Serves 8
1 Serving =
1 Fruit Exchange
½ Bread Exchange
1 Fat Exchange
120 Calories

C = 17.5 P = 1 F = 5

½ recipe pastry crust - baked - prepared for 1 crust pie

2 cups frozen unsweetened strawberries, blueberries or raspberries
1 cup unsweetened grape juice (red for strawberries & raspberries – White or Purple for blueberries)
1 envelope unflavored gelatin

Defrost berries but do not drain. Mash ½ cup berries to draw more juice and mix with remaining whole berries and berry liquid. Mix gelatin and grape juice in small sauce pan and let set 2 minutes. Bring to a boil stirring to dissolve gelatin. Mix juice/gelatin mix in berries. Let cool to room temperature and pour in shell. Refrigerate until set. Top with a dollop of whipped cream.

*This filling may also be used as a topping for custard, puddings or cheese cake.

BLUEBERRY-CREAM CHEESE PIE

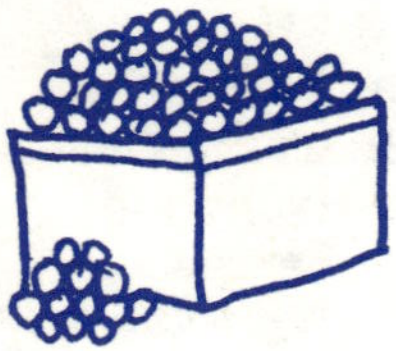

Serves 8
1 Serving Equals
3 Fat Exchanges
1 Fruit Exchange
½ Bread Exchange
½ Medium Fat Meat Exchange
245 Calories

C = 17.5 P = 4.5 F = 17.5

1 9 inch baked pastry shell (1 crust type)
1 1 pound can blueberries, juice or water pack
1 8-¾ ounce can crushed pineapple in pineapple juice
1 8 ounce package neufchatel cheese, room temperature
1 tablespoon milk
½ teaspoon vanilla
2 tablespoons cornstarch
dash of salt
½ teaspoon lemon juice
1 cup whipped cream

Drain fruits in separate bowls reserving juice. Blend neufchatel cheese, milk and vanilla. Stir in pineapple (reserve 2 tablespoons for garnish). Spread cheese-pineapple mixture in bottom of crust. Refrigerate. Measure pineapple juice and add enough blueberry liquid to equal 1-½ cups. Over medium heat stir juices, cornstarch and salt until thickened. Stir in blueberries and lemon juice. Cool. Pour over cheese layer. Chill. Top with whipped cream and garnish with reserved pineapple bits.

BLUEBERRY-PEACH PIE

Serves 8
1 Serving Equals
1-¼ Fruit Exchange
1 Bread Exchange
2 Fat Exchanges
210 Calories
C = 27.5 P = 2 F = 10

Pastry crust for 2 crust 9" pie
1 cup unsweetened blueberries – fresh or drained canned or frozen
16 ounce can sliced peaches canned in fruit juice, undrained
2-½-3 tablespoons tapioca
¾ teaspoon cinnamon

Preheat oven to 425°. Line bottom of pie plate with crust. Mix all filling ingredients. Pour into prepared bottom crust. Top with remaining crust. Seal edges. Cut slits (I like to make a tree shape) in top crust to allow steam to escape. Bake 40-50 minutes until golden brown. Remove from oven and cool on rack.

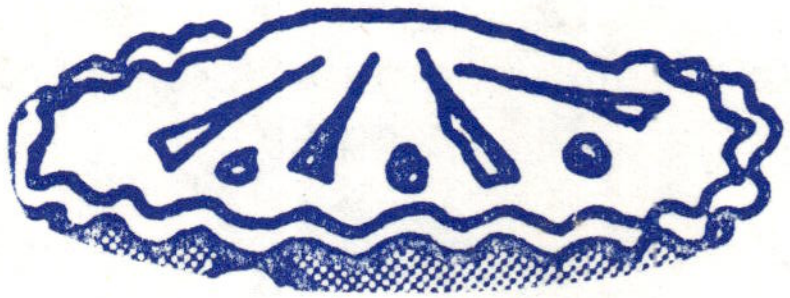

"WINTER" FRUIT PIE

Serves 8
1 Serving Equals
½ Bread Exchange
1 Fat Exchange
1-½ Fruit Exchange
140 Calories

C = 23 P = 1 F = 5

1 baked 8" pie shell, cooled
1 cup cooked apricots (about ¼ lb. dried)
1 cup cooked prunes (about ½ lb. dried)
1 cup apple juice
½ teaspoon cinnamon
2 tablespoons cornstarch

Cook apricots and prunes separately. Drain and remove pits. Mix cold juice, cinnamon and cornstarch in small sauce pan. Cook over medium heat until thickened. Stir in prunes and apricots. Cool to room temperature (keeps crust from getting soggy). Pour into baked crust. Refrigerate until serving time.

*Good plain or with a dollop of whipped or sour cream.

PIE CRUST

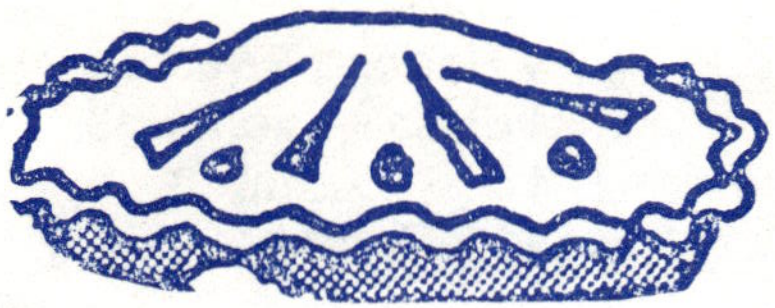

Serves 8
1 Serving (crust only) =
150 Calories
1 Bread Exchange
2 Fat Exchanges

C = 15 P = 2 F = 10

1 cup flour
dash of salt
⅓ cup shortening
2 tablespoons cold water

In a small bowl, mix flour and salt. Add shortening and cut into flour until particles are about the size of peas. Add water and mix with a fork until the dough forms a ball. Roll out on a lightly floured board or pastry canvas. If rolled very thin, makes enough for one 9 or 10 inch pie shell or an 8 inch 2 crust pie.

GRAHAM CRACKER CRUST

Serves 6
1 Serving Equals
1 Bread Exchange
1 Fat Exchange
115 Calories

12 graham crackers (squares)
2 tablespoons melted butter or margarine

C = 15 P = 2 F = 5

Crush graham crackers. Melt butter and mix with cracker crumbs. Press into 8 inch pie plate. Refrigerate 1 hour before filling with cool filling. Bake 7-8 minutes at 350° (until lightly brown and firm) allow to cool, if filling with warm filling.

*An easy way to crumb the crackers is in your blender or place crackers in large plastic baggie and roll with rolling pin until finely crushed.

GRAHAM CRACKER-WALNUT CRUST

Serves 6
1 Serving Equals
1 Bread Exchange
2 Fat Exchanges
160 Calories

1 cup graham cracker crumbs (12 squares)
7 teaspoons butter or margarine
⅓ cup finely chopped nuts

C = 15 P = 2 F = 10

Combine crumbs and nuts in 8 inch pie plate or spring form pan. Melt butter or margarine and mix with crumbs. Press into bottom or sides of pan. Refrigerate 1 hour allowing butter to chill and set crust. Fill as desired.

*Rich nutty flavor makes any dessert extra special.

SOUR CREAM ROLL UPS

Makes 48 cookies
2 Cookies Equal
⅔ Bread Exchange
2-½ Fat Exchange
⅓ Fruit Exchange
170 Calories

C = 14 P = 1 F = 12.5

2 cups flour
1 cup butter or margarine, room temperature
¾ cup sour cream
1 egg yolk
1 cup chopped dates
1 cup water
¾ cup chopped walnuts
1 tab grated orange peel

Cut soft butter or margarine into flour until mixture resembles corn meal. Add sour cream and egg yolk. Divide into 4 balls – wrap and refrigerate 2 hours. While dough chills combine dates and water in a sauce pan. Cook over medium heat until thick sauce forms. Remove from heat and stir in nuts and peel. Cool. To make cookies take one ball of chilled dough at a time and roll as for pie crust into a 10"-12" circle. Spread ¼ of filling on dough and cut into 12 pie shaped wedges. (I like to use a ravioli cutter for fancy edges). Roll each cookie from outside of circle to center and place point end down on ungreased cookie sheet. Bake in preheated 375° oven on top rack 20-25 minutes. Watch carefully as these brown easily. If browning too soon turn oven down a little or bake on double cookie sheet. Cool completely on wire racks. Cover and store in air tight tins.

*Flaky and tender
*Our all year round favorite.

MINI-COOKIE TARTS

Makes 24 cookies
2 Cookies Equals
3-⅓ Fat Exchanges
⅓ Medium Fat Meat
⅓ Fruit Exchange
⅔ Bread Exchange
215 Calories

C = 14 P = F = 18

½ cup butter or margarine, room temperature
1 3 ounce package cream cheese, room temperature
1-¼ cup flour
8 teaspoons apple juice concentrate
1 tablespoon butter or margarine, melted
1 cup chopped walnuts or pecans
¼ cup chopped dates
2 eggs, slightly beaten
½ teaspoon vanilla

Preheat oven to 350°. Mix butter cream cheese and flour to form soft dough. Make into 24 balls. Press 1 ball in each individual tart mold to form 1-½" inch shells. Set pastry shells aside. In small sauce pan melt butter over low heat. Remove pan from stove. Add apple juice concentrate, nuts, dates, and vanilla. Stir in beaten eggs, mix well. Spoon into unbaked prepared shells. Bake for 20-25 minutes until lighlty browned and puffy.

*Beautiful holiday cookies.
*Rich and flaky.

CHEESE COOKIES

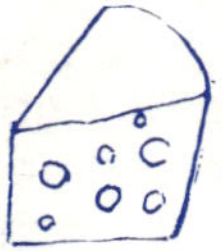

Makes 96 Cookies
2 Cookies Equals
½ Fat Exchange
1/6 Bread Exchange
⅓ High Fat Meat Exchange
70 Calories

C = 2.5 P = 3.0 F = 5

*Make holiday cookies with a cookie press.

½ cup butter or margarine, room temperature
½ cup shortening
4 cups cheddar cheese, finely grated
2-½ cups flour
½ teaspoon salt
½ teaspoon dry mustard
1 tablespoon chopped nuts

Preheat oven to 350°. With mixer cream butter and shortening until well mixed and fluffy. Beat in cheese. Add ½ cup flour, salt and dry mustard beating until well mixed. Add remaining flour 1 cup at a time. When well mixed fill cookie press (or gun) and form cookies following directions for press on ungreased cookie sheet. Use nut piece to garnish centers of flowers or sprinkle on ribbons. Bake 9-11 minutes for medium thick shapes, checking early for thin cookie shapes and bake only until beginning to brown on edge. Cool carefully on wire rack.

*A bit of coloring in dough makes interesting holiday cookies!

ALMOND ANGEL KISSES

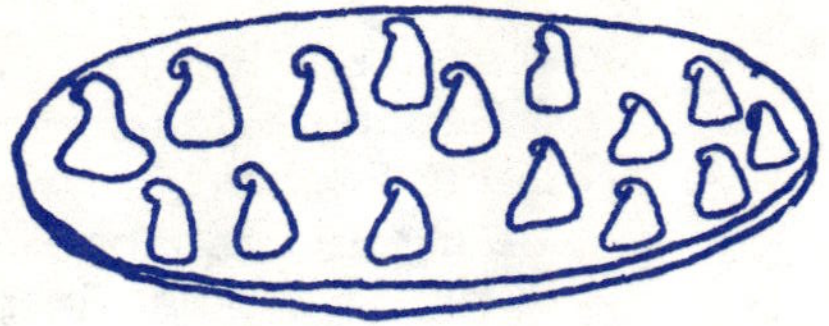

Makes 36 cookies
1 Cookie Equals
1 Fat Exchange
Fruit is negligible
50 Calories

C = 1 P = 0 F = 10

3 egg whites
¼ teaspoon cream of tartar
2 tablespoons apple juice concentrate
1 drop almond extract
1-½ cup ground almonds (unsalted)

Beat egg whites until foamy. Gradually add cream of tartar beating until stiff. Beat in apple juice concentrate. Add drop of extract. Gently fold in nuts. Drop by teaspoons to form kisses on cookie sheet lined with baking parchment. Bake at 325° until lightly browned 10-15 minutes. Cool completely before covering.

Walnuts and a dash of cinnamon may be substituted for almonds and extract.

APPLESAUCE BARS

Serves 8
1 Serving Equals
1 Fruit Exchange
2 Fat Exchange
1 Bread Exchange
200 Calories
C = 25 P = 2 F = 10

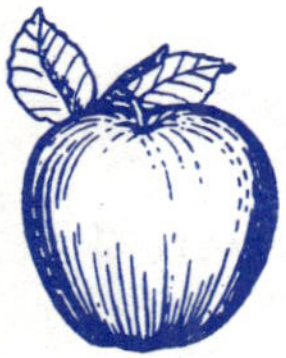

½ cup applesauce
½ cup apple juice
3 eggs
¼ cup butter or margarine
2 cups flour
½ teaspoon salt
1 teaspoon baking soda
2 teaspoons baking powder
½ teaspoon nutmeg
1-½ teaspoons cinnamon
¼ cup chopped nuts
¾ cup raisins

Preheat oven to 350°. Grease and flour an 8" square pan. In medium mixing bowl beat applesauce, apple juice, eggs and butter until well blended. Add flour, salt, baking soda, baking powder, nutmeg and cinnamon. Beat on medium speed 2 minutes, scraping sides often. Stir in nuts and raisins. Bake 25-30 minutes until a pick inserted in center comes out clean.

*Yummy with a dollop of whipped cream or topped with French pastry icing.

ORANGE-RAISIN DROP COOKIES

30 Cookies
2 Cookies Equals
1 Bread Exchange
1-½ Fat Exchange
Fruit Negligible
145 Calories
C = 17 P = 2 F = 7.5

1-¾ cups flour
2 teaspoons baking powder
¼ teaspoon salt
½ teaspoon cinnamon
¾ cup orange juice
½ teaspoon grated orange rind (if desired for a more distinct orange flavor)
7 tablespoons vegetable oil
1 egg
½ cup chopped walnuts or pecans
½ cup raisins

Preheat oven to 375°. Combine all ingredients and mix well. Drop by heaping teaspoons onto ungreased – no stick – cookie sheet. Bake 12-15 minutes until firm and lightly brown. Cool on wire rack.

REFRIGERATOR COOKIES

Makes 64 Cookies
1 Fat Exchange
½ Fruit Exchange
¼ Bread Exchange
83 Calories
2 cookies
C = 9 P = .5 F = 5

½ cup butter or margarine
1 egg
2 teaspoons vanilla
1 teaspoon baking powder
dash of salt
1 cup flour
1 cup chopped-unsugared dates
1 cup shredded coconut
1 cup chopped walnuts or pecans

Cream butter, egg and vanilla until mixed and fluffy. Beat in dry ingredients gradually mixing well after each addition. Mix in dates, coconut and ½ cup nuts. Form dough into two 1-½ inch logs. Roll logs in remaining nuts (¼ cup each). Wrap in waxed paper and chill (or freeze) until firm enough to slice. Preheat oven to 350°. Slice cookies ¼"-⅜" thick and place on non stick cookie sheet. Bake 10-12 minutes until light golden brown. Cool on wire racks.

JIFFY PEACH COBBLER

1 16 ounce can sliced peaches in fruit juice
2 teaspoons tapioca
cinnamon to taste
1 cup biscuit mix
⅓ cup milk

Serves 6
1 Serving =
110 Calories
1 Bread Exchange
1 Fruit Exchange

C = 25 P = 2 F = 0

Preheat oven to 350°. Combine peaches and juice, tapioca and cinnamon in a 9" pie plate. Stir together biscuit mix and milk in small bowl and top fruit with 6 equal sized "mounds" of biscuit dough.

Bake 25-30 minutes.

Serve warm with fruit dished on top of biscuit.
*Garnish with dollop of whipped cream if desired.
*Great breakfast treat
*Quick dessert that cooks while eating dinner!

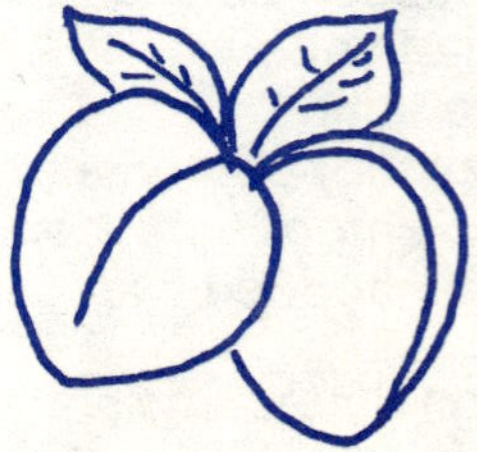

JIFFY APRICOT COBBLER

Substitute 1 16 ounce can apricots for peaches and add 1 drop of almond extract. Values are the same as with peaches.

CRAZY COBBLER

Serves 6
1 Serving Equals
1 Bread Exchange
1 Fruit Exchange
½ Fat Exchange
135 Calories

C = 25 P = 2 F = 2.5

1 16 ounce can fruit cocktail in fruit juice
2 teaspoons tapioca
½ teaspoon cinnamon
1 cup biscuit mix
⅓ cup milk
3 tablespoons chopped nuts

Preheat oven to 350°.
Combine fruit cocktail and juice, tapioca, cinnamon and nuts in a 9" pie plate. In small bowl stir together biscuit mix and milk. Drop biscuit dough on fruit in 6 equal mounds. Bake 25-30 minutes. Serve warm.

*Good with milk or cream at breakfast.
*Add a dollop of whipped cream and dessert in a jiffy!

ORANGE DATE SNACKIN' CAKE

Makes 1 small loaf
12 Slices
1 Slice =
135 Calories
½ Fruit Exchange
1 Fat Exchange
1 Bread Exchange

C = 25 P = 2 F = 5

9 large pitted dates, chopped to make about ½ cup
½ cup non fat dry milk
¼ cup butter or stick-type margarine, softened
1 egg
¾ cup orange juice
1 cup flour
1-½ teaspoons baking powder
½ teaspoon salt

Cream butter or margarine with dry milk powder. Add egg and orange juice and beat well. Stir in flour, baking powder and salt. Mix until well blended. Stir in chopped dates, mixing well until evenly distributed.

Preheat oven to 325°. Bake in a lightly greased loaf pan for 45-50 minutes, until cake appears done and a wooden toothpick inserted in center comes out clean. Cool and slice.

*This is a heavy type cake and is good in lunches as it can be eaten easily with fingers.

CARROT CAKE

Serves 14
1 Serving equals
1 Bread Exchange
1 Vegetable Exchange
½ Fruit Exchange
1-½ Fat Exchange
185 Calories

C = 25 P = 4 F = 7.5

½ cup butter or margarine, room temperature
3 eggs
1 cup unsweetened pineapple juice
2-½ cups flour
1 teaspoon baking soda
2 teaspoons baking powder
½ teaspoon salt
1 teaspoon nutmeg
1-½ teaspoons cinnamon
3 cups grated carrots
1 cup unsweetened crushed pineapple, drained

Preheat oven to 350°. Lightly grease and flour 9 x 13 baking pan and set aside. Cream eggs and butter. Stir in pineapple juice. Add remaining ingredients except carrot and pineapple and beat 2 minutes. Stir in carrots and **well** drained pineapple. Pour into pan and spread out evenly. Bake 30-35 minutes until center springs back lightly when touched and cake is lightly browned. Cool on wire rack.

*Excellent frosted with cream cheese or French pastry icing.

PINEAPPLE UPSIDE DOWN CAKE

Serves 9
1 Serving Equals
1 Bread Exchange
¾ Fruit Exchange
1 Fat Exchange
145 Calories

C = 22 P = 2 F = 5

Topping:
1 20 ounce can crushed juice packed pineapple, drained – reserve juice
¾ teaspoon cinnamon or nutmeg
1 tablespoon melted butter or margarine

Cake:
1-½ cup flour
½ teaspoon baking soda
1 teaspoon baking powder
½ cup reserved pineapple juice
2 tablespoons milk
1 egg
¼ cup oil

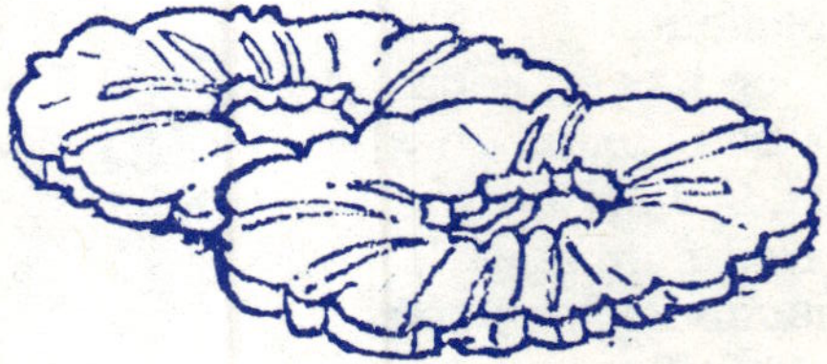

Preheat oven to 350°. Lightly grease 8" square or 8" round cake dish. Melt butter and mix with well drained pineapple and spice. Spread evenly in bottom of pan. Combine flour, baking powder, baking soda in mixing bowl. Add egg, oil, milk and pineapple juice and beat well. Pour batter over pineapple. Bake 28-30 minutes. Cool about 15 minutes (will still be warm) and carefully invert onto serving plate. Serve warm with whipped cream.

*2 tablespoons whipped cream equals 1 fat exchange, 45 calories, C = 0 P = 0 F = 5.

PINEAPPLE COFFEE-CAKE

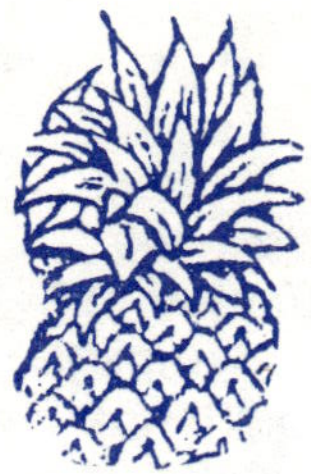

Serves 12
1 Serving equals
1 Bread Exchange
1 Fruit Exchange
1 Fat Exchange
155 Calories

C = 25 P = 2 F = 5

¼ cup butter or margarine
2 eggs
⅔ cup unsweetened pineapple juice
2 cups flour
½ teaspoon baking soda
2 teaspoons baking powder
½ teaspoon salt
1-½ cups juice packed crushed pineapple, drained
1 cup unsweetened shredded or flaked coconut
½ teaspoon cinnamon
¼ cup chopped walnuts

Preheat oven to 350°. Lightly grease and flour a 9 inch square baking pan and set aside. Cream together eggs, butter and pineapple juice. Add flour, baking soda, baking powder and salt. Beat 2 minutes. Gently mix in 1 cup of drained, crushed pineapple and coconut. Pour into prepared pan. Sprinkle remaining pineapple over top. Mix nuts and cinnamon and top cake batter. Bake approximately 25 minutes until center springs back when lightly touched and cake is golden.

Yummy warm with a dollop of whipped cream!

SPICY BANANA-NUT CAKE

Serves 12
1 Serving equals
1 Bread Exchange
½ Fruit Exchange
2-½ Fat Exchange
205 Calories

C = 20 P = 2 F = 125

½ cup butter or margarine, room temperature
3 small ripe bananas (about 1 cup)
3 eggs
¾ cup water
2 cups flour
2 teaspoons baking powder
1 teaspoon baking soda
¼ teaspoon salt
¾ teaspoon cinnamon
¾ cup chopped walnuts

Preheat oven to 350°. Lightly grease and flour 9 x 13 pan and set aside.

Mash bananas in large mixing bowl and mix with butter or margarine. Add eggs and water mixing well. Mix in flour, baking powder, baking soda, salt, and cinnamon until smooth. Stir in chopped nuts. Pour into prepared pan. Bake 20-25 minutes until wooden pick inserted in center comes out clean.

*Excellent with French pastry icing or a dollop of whipped cream.

*Orange French pastry icing makes a delightful flavor combination.

APPLE FRITTERS

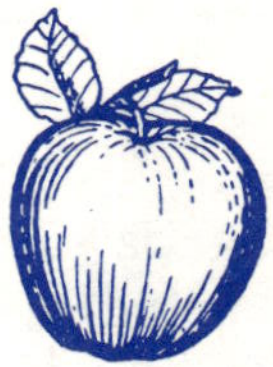

(Fruit Filled Drop Doughnuts)

Makes 16
1 Fritter Equals
½ Bread Exchange
¼ Fruit Exchange
½ Fat Exchange
68 Calories

C = 10 P = 1 F = 2.5

1 cup flour, unsifted
1-¼ teaspoon baking powder
1 teaspoon salt
½ teaspoon cinnamon, nutmeg or apple pie spice
2 eggs
6 tablespoons milk
2 tablespoons apple juice concentrate
1 teaspoon vegetable oil
1 apple, peeled and chopped, core removed

Combine first four dry ingredients in mixing bowl and set aside. In small bowl mix eggs, milk, concentrate and oil. Beat until smooth. Add apple bits. Drop by tablespoonsful into hot 375° fat and fry until golden brown. Drain on paper towels. Serve warm.

PINEAPPLE FRITTERS

Substitute 1 cup well drained juice packed crushed pineapple for the chopped apple. Values same as apple fritters.

CREAM PUFFS

Makes 6
1 Puff Equals
½ Bread Exchange
½ Medium Fat Meat Exchange
1-½ Fat Exchange
125 Calories

C = 7.5 P = 4.5 F = 9

½ cup water
¼ cup butter
½ cup flour
2 eggs

Heat water and butter to rolling boil in saucepan. Stir in flour and keep stirring until mixture forms a ball. Remove from heat and beat in eggs one at a time. Beat until smooth. Drop from spoon on ungreased cookie sheet. Bake at 400° approximately 40 minutes. Shells should be puffed, dry and golden brown.

Cool away from drafts. Cut off tops and remove soft centers. Fill as desired.

*These are yummy when filled with whipped cream. For a special occasion sometimes fill them with a scoop of ice cream and top with chocolate sauce or strawberry topping.

*Custards and fruit creams are also favorite fillings.

CREAM PUFF SWANS

Make cream puffs above but reserve a small amount of batter to shape in 6 2" S shapes. Bake "S"'s with shells. When cool and filling shells insert one S per puff for head. Fill and top with lid split for wings.

CREAM PUFF WREATH

Serves 12
Values same as cream
puff servings.

Make double cream puff recipe taking care to beat all 4 eggs in one at a time. Place in a circle on ungreased baking sheet with the 12 mounds about 1-½ – 1-¾ inches apart. Bake as directed. Dough will puff and edges touch. Carefully slit top off entire ring and fill as desired. Trim wreath with ribbon – holly – or pine boughs. Really a dessert-centerpiece in one!

*Good with a strawberry chiffon filling or berries folded in whipped cream.

CUSTARD FILLING

Serves 6
1 Serving Equals
⅓ Milk Exchange
½ Medium Fat Meat Exchange
½ Fruit Exchange
65 Calories
C = 9 P = 4 F = 1.5

4 tab cornstarch
2 cups skim milk
3 egg yolks
2 teaspoons vanilla
4 tablespoons apple juice concentrate, defrosted

Combine all ingredients. Cook over medium heat until mix thickens, stirring occasionally. Cool before filling desserts.

*Also makes good base for fruit topping and fruit parfaits.

FRESH STRAWBERRY SHORTCAKE

Serves 4
1 Serving Equals
1-½ Fruit Exchange
1 Bread Exchange
1 Fat Exchange
175 Calories

C = 30 P = 2 F = 5

3 cups fully ripe strawberries
½ cup unsweetened white grape juice or 8 teaspoons apple juice concentrate
4 2" diameter baking powder biscuits
½ cup whipped cream with vanilla to taste.

Wash and slice or mash berries (leaving 4 whole for garnish). Mix the grape juice with the berries. Split the biscuits and spoon half the berries in the center – replace the top and add remaining berries. Top each shortcake with 2 tablespoons whipped cream. Garnish with whole ripe berry.

*Apple juice concentrate is sweeter..
*White grape juice provides more juice.

RASPBERRY SHORTCAKE

Substitute 2 cups of fresh raspberries for strawberries.

ORANGE CREAM DESSERT

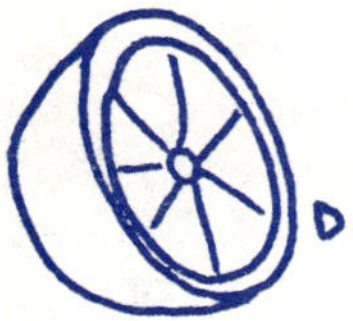

Serves 8
1 Serving =
½ Fruit Exchange
2 Fat Exchange
125 Calories

C = 5 P = 0 F = 10

2 cups unsweetened orange juice
1 envelope unflavored gelatin
1 drop almond extract
1 cup whipping cream

Mix gelatin and ½ cup orange juice in small bowl and let set 2 minutes to soften. Boil remaining juice and add to gelatin mix and stir until dissolved. Refrigerate until thick and syrupy. Beat cream until light and fluffy. Add 1 drop almond to whipped cream and slowly add gelatin mixture cream until just blended. Spoon into individual dessert dishes and refrigerate until set.

*May be refrigerated in a ring mold. Unmold and serve on platter with drained mandarin or fresh orange slices for garnish.

*Rich, elegant and tastes like the "old fashioned" cream-sicle!

QUICK APPLE (PLUM) DESSERT

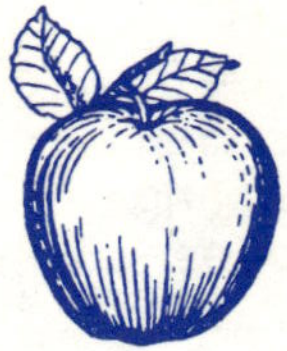

Serves 9
1 Serving Equals
1 Bread Exchange
1-½ Fruit Exchange
130 Calories

C = 30 P = 2 F = 0

*If desired – 1 tablespoon whipped cream per serving adds 25 calories – 2.5 g. fat.

2 cups fully ripe plums, pitted and chopped
2 medium apples, sliced and peeled
¼ cup apple juice concentrate
2 tablespoons cornstarch or tapioca
¼ teaspoon cinnamon
1-½ cups biscuit mix
½ cup skim milk

Mix plums, apples, apple juice concentrate, cinnamon and cornstarch or tapioca in 8" square pan. Mix milk and biscuit mix and drop in 9 equal mounds on fruit. Bake at 350° for 30-40 minutes until biscuits are lightly brown and fruit is tender and thickened.

Delicious warm with a tablespoon of whipped cream.

Pretty served in wine or stem type glasses.

Great for dessert or a real brunch treat.

SPICY CINNAMON PEAR TWISTS

Topping
2 teaspoons melted butter
1 teaspoon cinnamon
3 tablespoons apple pear concentrate
5 tablespoons boiling water

2 fresh pears
1-½ cup flour
½ cup shortening
dash of salt
3 to 4 tablespoons cold water (for dough)

Serves 8
1 Serving Equals
(2 twists)
1-½ Bread Exchange
3 Fat Exchange
½ Fruit Exchange
285 Calories

C = 28 P = 3 F = 15

Preheat oven to 450°. Wash and core pears. Cut each pear into 8 slices. Set aside. Mix flour and salt in bowl. Add shortening and cut into flour until the size of peas. Add water and mix into a ball. Divide dough in half and roll each half out on a lightly floured pastry canvas into an 8 x 10 inch rectangle. Cut each rectangle into 8 (10" x 1") strips. Wrap one strip of dough around each pear wedge. Place in a 9 x 13 baking pan without touching. Brush with melted butter to which cinnamon was added. Mix water and concentrate and pour around pastries. Bake at 20-25 minutes until golden brown.

*Excellent served warm with milk or cream.

SPICY CINNAMON APPLE TWISTS

Substitute apples for pears and apple juice concentrate for apple-pear concentrate. Values remain the same as using pears.

PARADISE PIE

Serves 8
1 Serving Equals
½ Bread Exchange
2 Fat Exchanges
1-½ Fruit Exchanges
185 Calories

C = 22.5 P = 1 F = 10

Crust
½ recipe pastry crust (page 63)

Filling
1 orange, peeled and chopped
1 20 oz. can crushed pineapple in pineapple juice
2 tablespoons tapioca or cornstarch
5 tablespoons light or golden raisins

Topping
1 cup whipped cream

Prepare pastry crust for 1 crust pie – pricking bottom and sides with fork. Bake in 425° oven 7-8 minutes until lightly browned. Remove from oven and allow to cool. Combine filling ingredients in medium sauce pan. Simmer oven, low heat, stirring occasionally, until mixture thickens (20-25 minutes). Cool to room temperature and pour into cooled pastry shell. Chill and top with whipped cream.

*Cream may be flavored with a drop of orange extract or pineapple flavoring, if desired.

PINEAPPLE "CHEATCAKE"

(A cheesecake with too few calories to believe!)
No crust – low calorie

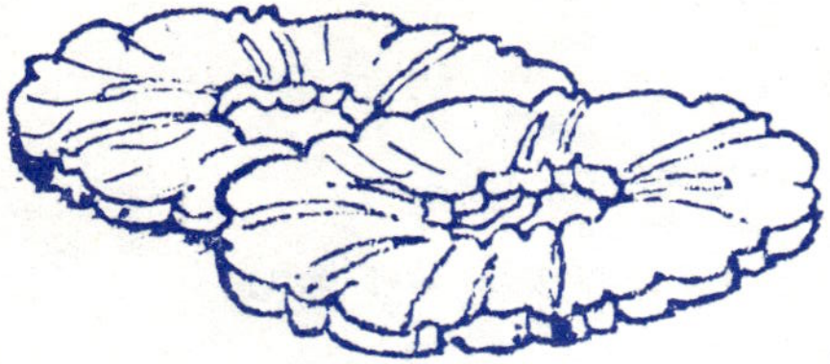

Serves 8
1 Serving Equals
1 Fruit Exchange
1 Fat Exchange
½ Medium Fat Meat Exchange
Milk Negligible
125 Calories

C = 10 P = 40 F = 7.5

1 20 ounce can pineapple in juice
1 envelope unflavored gelatin
½ cup skim milk
1 8 ounce packageNeufchatel(cream-type) cheese
1 teaspoon vanilla
¼ teaspoon lemon juice
2 egg whites

Drain pineapple and reserve one cup of juice. (If there is not one cup add water to make one cup.) In a small sauce pan mix gelatin and milk. Cook over low heat about 2 minutes, stirring constantly, to dissolve gelatin completely. Remove from heat. In a large mixing bowl beat cheese until smooth and fluffy. Gradually beat in hot gelatin/milk mixture blending well. Next beat in the one cup pineapple juice, vanilla and lemon juice. Chill until mixture holds a kiss shape when dropped from a spoon. (about ½ hour). Beat egg whites until stiff. Fold egg whites and drained pineapple bits into cheese filling mixture. Turn into a 9 inch pieplate or spring form pan and chill until firm – 3 to 4 hours.

STUFFED DATES

Serves 16
1 Serving Equals
1 Fruit Exchange
Fat negligible
20 Calories

C = 10 P = 0 F = 0

16 medium pitted dates, non sugared
¼ cup flaked coconut, unsweetened
8 walnut halves

Break walnut halves in half. 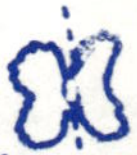 forming two long sections per half. Stuff 1 nut section into each date. Roll in coconut. Place in a pretty candy dish. Enjoy!

*Coconut may be colored to accent a special holiday season or occasion. Simply mix in small plastic baggie with a small amount of food coloring and work with hands before coating dates.

*These go back to my childhood. I can remember making these for gifts and proudly presenting them as one of my first "cooking" projects.

*Small soft dried prunes may be substituted for dates.

CREAM CHEESE BON BONS

Makes 16 Bon Bons
1 Serving Equals
1-½ Fat Exchange
¼ Medium Fat Meat Exchange
⅛ Fruit Exchange
Milk – negligible
102 Calories

C = 3 P = 3 F = 8.75

1 8 ounce package neufchatel cheese, room temperature
1 teaspoon almond extract
4 teaspoons apple-pear concentrate, defrosted
8 teaspoons skim milk powder
1 cup chopped nuts

Mix cheese, extract concentrate and skim milk powder. Roll into 16 balls and roll in nuts to coat. Refrigerate until firm. Store refrigerated.

COCONUT CREAM CONFECTIONS

Makes 16
1 Serving Equals 2 Candies
1 Fat Exchange
⅔ Fruit Exchange
¼ Medium Fat Exchange
Milk – negligible
90 Calories

C = 7 P = 2 F = 6.25

½ 8 oz. package Neufchatel cheese
¼ cup apple-pear concentrate, defrosted
1 cup shredded or flaked coconut, unsweetened
¼ teaspoon almond extract
4 tablespoons instant milk powder

Mix all ingredients and form into 16 little balls. Refrigerate until serving.

*At Easter color the coconut and mold into egg shapes.

FROZEN YOGURT POPS

Makes 8 Pops
1 Pop Equals
¼ Milk Exchange
1 Fruit Exchange
60 Calories

C = 13 P = 2 F = 0

2 8 ounce cartons plain yogurt
6 ounce frozen fruit concentrate

Slush concentrate in blender. Add yogurt and blend until smooth. Pour into 3 ounce paper cups and place in freezer. When partially set insert sticks. Freeze firmly. Enjoy!

*Grape is a favorite . . . purple and sweet!

BASIC SWEET "GUMDROP" CHEW

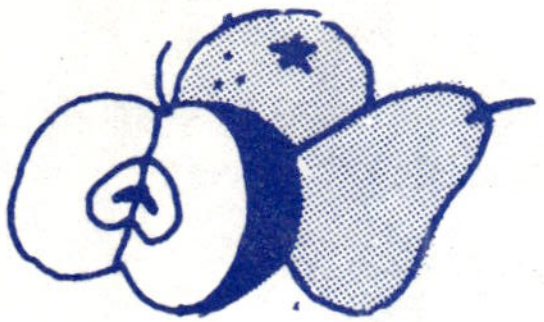

Apple Chews – 4 Squares
Grape Chews – 3 Squares
Orange Chews – 5 Squares
Equal ½ Fruit Exchange
10 Calories

C = 5 P = 0 F = 0

3 cups apple juice, grape juice or orange juice
5 envelopes gelatin

Soften gelatin in 1 cup fruit juice in medium mixing bowl. Bring 1 cup juice to a boil and stir in gelatin/juice mix. Continue stirring until gelatin is dissolved. Add remaining cup of juice. Pour into 8" square pan and refrigerate until firm. Cut into 1" squares to serve.

*Red grape juice makes great chews.
*For a festive touch – cut squares with cookie cutter into holiday shapes – orange pumpkins – red hearts, etc.

"GUMDROP" FRUIT CHEWS

Makes 64 Squares
3 Squares Equals
¼ Fruit Exchange
5 Calories

$C = 2.5$ $P = 0$ $F = 0$

Orange Pineapple Chews
4 envelopes gelatin
1 cup canned unsweetened pineapple juice
1 cup orange juice
¾ cup boiling water

In medium bowl mix gelatin with pineapple juice. Let rest 2 minutes to soften gelatin. Add boiling water and stir until gelatin is dissolved. Stir in cold orange juice. Pour into 8 inch pan and chill until firm. Cut into 1" squares to serve.

GRANOLA BARS

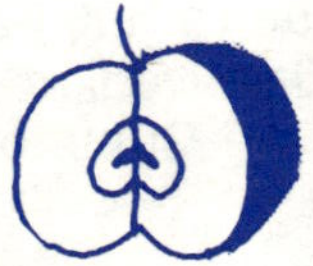

Serves 8
2 Bars Equal
2 Fruit Exchanges
¼ Bread Exchange
1 Fat Exchange
145 Calories

$C = 24$ $P = .5$ $F = 5$

2-⅔ cups apple juice
2 cups granola
5 envelopes gelatin

Soften gelatin in ⅔ cup juice in mixing bowl. Boil one cup juice and stir in gelatin/juice. Continue stirring until gelatin dissolves. Add remaining cup of juice and stir in granola. Pour into 8" saucepan. Chill until set. Cut into 16 bars.

*Great for snacks, picnics or lunch boxes.
*Quick energy on the go!

APPLE-NUT SQUARES

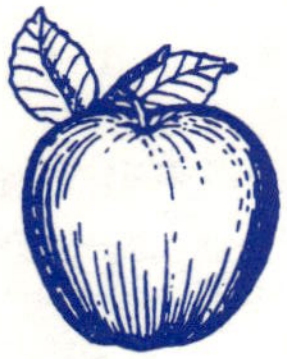

Serves 8
1 Serving Equals
1 Fruit Exchange
1 Fat Exchange
95 Calories

C = 10 P = 0 F = 5

1 6 ounce can unsweetened apple juice concentrate, thawed
½ cup boiling water
3 envelopes unflavored gelatin
½ cup chopped walnuts or pecans

Place half apple juice concentrate in small bowl with gelatin. Let rest one minute to soften gelatin. Stir in boiling water mixing until gelatin is dissolved. Add remaining juice and nuts. Pour into a loaf pan and chill until firm. Cut into 16 bars. Store in refrigerator.

*These crunchy little candy squares with a gum drop consistency stay firm for a lunch box treat.
*Nuts will be mostly on top. For nuts mixed throughout refrigerate juice/gelatin mix. and stir in nuts.

CHEESE BALL

Serves 8
1 Serving Equals
½ Medium Fat Meat Exchange
1-½ Fat Exchange
½ Fruit Exchange
Vegetable negligible
125 Calories
C = 5 P = 3.5 F = 10

2 8 ounce packages Neufchatel cheese
1 8-½ ounce can crushed pineapple (in juice type) drained
¼ cup chopped green pepper
2 tablespoons chopped sweet onion
1 tablespoon Beau Monde spice (Spice Island)
1 cup chopped nuts

Mix all ingredients except nuts. Divide into two balls. Chill 30 minutes for easier handling. Roll in nuts. Serve one now, freeze the other for a special occasion!

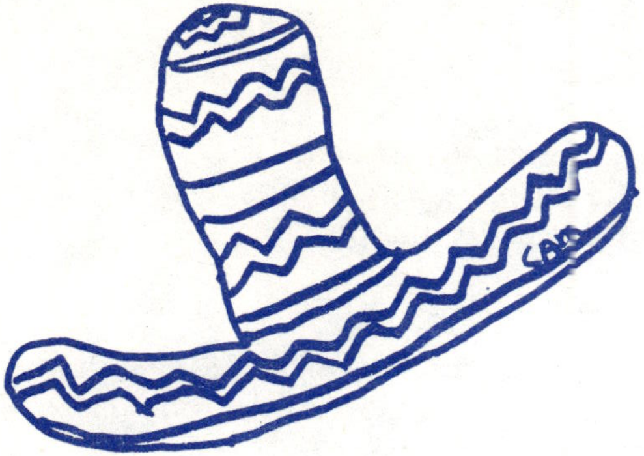

BEAN DIP

Makes 2 quarts/
Serves 36
1-¼ Cup Serving =
95 Calories
¾ High Fat Meat Exchange
¼ Bread Exchange
Negligible fruit and vegetable exchange

½ pound extra-lean ground beef
1 16 ounce can refried beans
1 8 ounce can tomato sauce
1 pound processed cheese (Velveeta type)
2 tablespoons (½ small can) chopped green chilies

Brown meat and drain off excess fat. Add remaining ingredients, stirring over low heat until cheese melts. Serve warm. This dip will freeze well.

Each ¼ cup serving equals ¾ high fat meat exchange; ¼ bread exchange; negligible fruit and vegetable exchanges; 95 calories.

*A favorite party snack for teens and men. Makes super nachos.
*Terrific burrito filling!

TORTILLA CHIPS

8 Pieces = 1 Serving
1 Serving = 70 Calories
1 Bread Exchange

1 package corn tortillas
salt

C = 15 P = 2 F = 0

Cut each tortilla into 8 pie shaped wedges. Spread the pieces on a cookie sheet and sprinkle lightly with salt. Bake them at 400° for about 8 minutes. Remove from the oven and with tongs or a pancake turner turn each one over. Bake for 3-4 more minutes. Cool on paper towels. Great with dips, salads and for a crunchy snack! A fat-free munchy.

Taco flavored seasoning gives a flavor of Old Mexico. Sometimes I use it instead of salt.

POPCORN

Corn popped in an air popper pops without fat and contains only 70 calories in 3 cups popped and C = 15 grams, protein = 2 grams and fat = 0. Popcorn is satisfying and provides good bulk and roughage. Toppings are what makes good popcorn great.

The following toppings sprinkled on popped corn are "free" and add nothing but flavor to your snack.

garlic salt	taco seasoning	butter-flavored salt	bacon-flavored salt
curry powder	dried Italian herbs	dill weed	herb tea leaves (finely crushed)
celery salt	hickory flavored salt	seasoned salt	herb tea salt
chili powder	vegetable flakes	powdered orange rind	caraway seeds

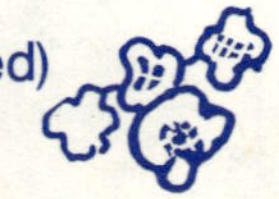

SNACKERS MIX

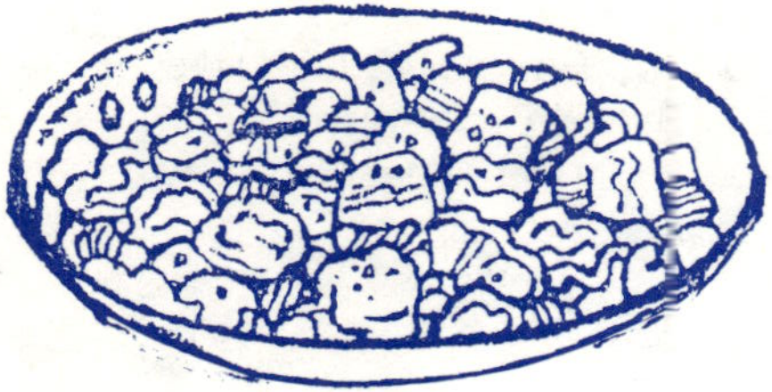

Makes 16 cups
1 Cup Equals
⅓ Bread Exchange
1 Fat Exchange
1 Fruit Exchange
110 Calories

C = 15 P = 1 F = 5

3 quarts popped popcorn
1 cup salted nuts
1 cup raisins
1 cup fresh shredded coconut (not sugared)
1 cup sunflower seeds

Pop corn without fat and allow to cool. Mix in remaining ingredients. Store in airtight container.

*This is good to pack in 1 cup amounts in individual sandwich bags for camper and hiking snacks. Goes great in a back-pack!

*Super idea for classroom snack treats.

KIDS SNACKIN CORN

1 Cup Equals 70 Calories
⅓ Bread Exchange
⅓ High Fat Meat Exchange
⅓ Fat Exchange

C = 5 P = 3 F = 5

9 cups popped corn
1 tablespoon butter or margarine
⅓ cup peanut butter

Pop the corn. This recipe is calculated on corn popped in an air type popper without added fat for fewer calories.

Over low heat melt the butter or margarine with peanut butter until runny. Drizzle over the popped corn and mix well. Spread in shallow baking pans and bake in 375 degree oven for 10 minutes stirring 2 or 3 times. The corn will crisp and topping will set.

Cool and enjoy.
Good for lunch crunchies and snacks.
Makes 9 cups.

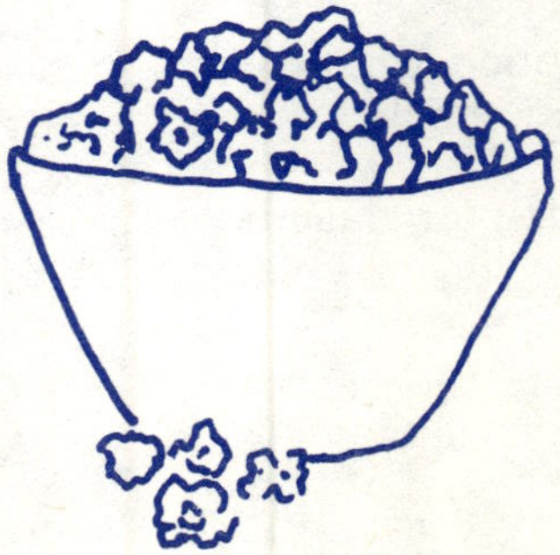

NIBBLE MIX

Serves 8
1 Serving Equals
1 Bread Exchange
2 Fat Exchanges
160 Calories

C = 15 P = 2 F = 10

2 quarts popped corn
2 cups thin pretzel sticks
2 cups baked cheese korn-type curls
¼ cup butter or margarine
1 tablespoon worcestershire sauce
¾ teaspoon garlic salt

Preheat over to 250°. In 9 x 13 baking dish mix popped corn, pretzels and cheese curls. Melt butter in small saucepan adding worcestershire sauce and garlic salt. Drizzle over popped corn mix and stir well. Bake 45 minutes stirring 5 times to mix during cooking time.

*Store leftovers – cool – in airtight containers.

FRUIT YOGURT

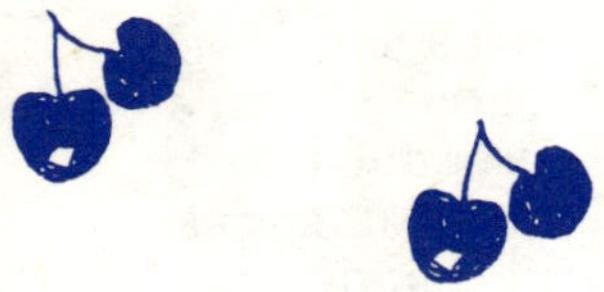

Serves 2
1 Serving = 60 Calories
½ Milk Exchange
½ Fruit Exchange

C = 11 P = 4 F = 0

1 8 ounce carton plain yogurt
½ cup raspberries, boysenberries, pitted cherries, peaches or pineapple

Wash and drain fresh berries (or drain frozen berries). Squish one half of fruit with potato masher and stir into yogurt. Add the remaining whole berries and mix gently – divide into two dishes and enjoy! Great for breakfast or dessert.

*Don't use the mixer as yogurt will get a bit watery if over mixed.

Serves 2
1 Serving = 80 Calories
½ Milk Exchange
1 Fruit Exchange

C = 16 P = 4 F = 0

A BIT OUT OF THE ORDINARY . . . stir ½ cup grape halves in yogurt and sprinkle with a dash of nutmeg.

PEANUT BUTTER 'n BANANAS

Serves 4
⅓ Cup Servings
1 Serving Equals
½ Fruit Exchange
⅛ Milk Exchange
1 High Fat Meat Exchange
½ Fat Exchange
125 Calories

C = 6.5 P = 8 F = 7.5

1 small ripe banana, mashed
½ cup plain non-fat yogurt
½ cup peanut butter, creamy
2 drops vanilla

Put all ingredients in blender and blend just until smooth but not watery. Place in individual dessert dishes and chill thoroughly.

*A favorite of children.
*For a quick snack put in small paper cups to chill.
*Freeze in hot weather for an icy treat.

GRANOLA

Makes 4 Cups
¼ Cup Equals
¼ Bread Exchange
1 Fat Exchange
1 Fruit Exchange
105 Calories

C = 14 P = .5 F = 5

1 cup rolled oats
½ cup coarsley chopped nuts
1 cup flaked or shredded unsweetened coconut
1 cup raisins
½ cup sunflower seeds

Mix all ingredients together and store in airtight container.

*½ cup chopped unsweetened dates may be substituted for ½ cup of the raisins.

*Super snack for the great outdoors!

SPARKLING APPLE "BUBBLY"

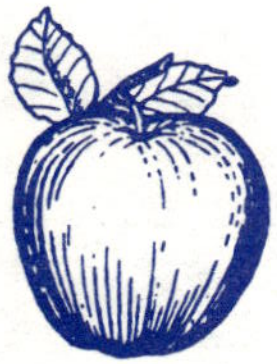

Serves 6
1 Serving Equals
1 Fruit Exchange
40 Calories

C = 10 P = 0 F = 0

2 cups unsweetened apple juice, well chilled
2 cups (16 ounce) club soda, well chilled

Combine the chilled apple juice and soda. Serve in frosted or chilled wine glasses.

LOW CALORIE STRAWBERRY SLUSH

Serves
1 Serving Equals
½ Fruit Exchange
20 Calories

C = 50 P = 0 F = 0

⅓ cup sliced strawberries
⅔ cup crushed ice
soda water

Whirl berries with any juice and ice in blender. Pour into a tall glass and stir in soda water to taste.

It's a wonderful refresher – quick and thirst quenching.

PARTY FRUIT PUNCH

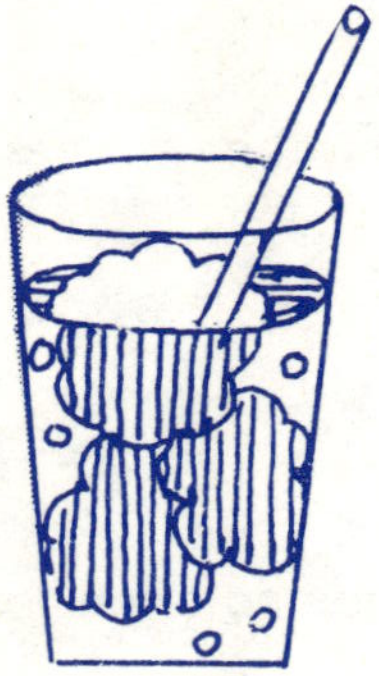

Makes 6 servings
Tall glasses
1 Serving Equals
40 Calories
1 Fruit Exchange

C = 10 P = 0 F = 0

or 12 ½ punch cups
1 Serving Equals
½ Fruit Exchange
20 Calories

C = 5 P = 0 F = 0

1 cup unsweetened orange juice
¾ cup white grape juice
⅓ cup pineapple juice
1 quart club soda (or 28 ounce bottle)

Combine all ingredients and serve over ice. Festive garnished with a mint sprig and tall straw.

*If using a punch bowl make ice in a ring mold and freeze fruit slices or flowers inside.

*Carbonation stays "fizzier" if juices and soda are chilled before mixing.

LEMONADE

1 cup fresh lemon juice
1-¾ cups unsweetened grape juice
(white juice for regular lemonade)
(red juice for "pink" lemonade)
¼ cup water

Makes 9 servings
1 Serving Equals
40 Calories
1 Fruit Exchange

C = 10 P = 0 F = 0

Mix lemon and grape juice with ¼ cup water. Refrigerate. Shake. Add ⅓ cup mix to 1 cup cold water. Add ice cubes. Garnish with lemon slices.

SPICED CIDER

2-⅔ cups apple cider
1-⅓ cups water
1 cinnamon stick
½ teaspoon whole cloves
½ teaspoon whole allspice
Orange and lemon slices for garnish
Cinnamon sticks (optional)

Makes 4 cups (8 servings)
½ cup =
40 Calories
1 Fruit Exchange

C = 10 P = 0 F = 0

Simmer cider, water and spices together in saucepan for 10 minutes. Strain, if spices were not put in garni bag. Serve hot with fruit slice garnish and cinnamon sticks, if desired.

*In punch bowl, top with baked clove-studded oranges.

ENJOY!

REAL GRAPE "POP"

Serves 1
12 Ounce Serving Equals
1 Fruit Exchange
40 Calories

C = 10 P = 0 F = 0

¼ cup purple or red grape juice
1 cup (8 oz.) club soda

Stir juice and club soda until mixed. (Take care not to over mix and loose carbonation) Pour over ice or mix in a glass with ice cubes.

REAL ORANGE "POP"

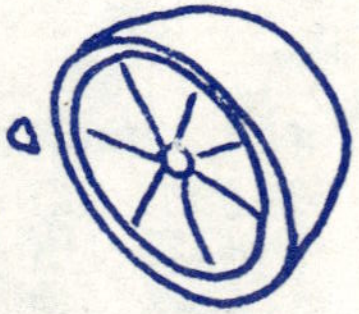

Serves 1
Equals 40 Calories
1 Fruit Exchange

C = 10 P = 0 F = 0

2 tablespoons orange juice concentrate
1 cup (8 oz. club soda)

Stir the juice concentrate until defrosted in botton of tall glass. Add club soda and ice. Enjoy!

*This is an excellent way to use juice drained off canned or frozen fruit. A drop of food coloring may be necessary to color if fruit was done in white grape juice.

VIRGIN MARY

Serves 2
1 Serving Equals
1 Vegetable Exchange
25 Calories

1 cup tomato juice
dash worcestershire sauce
dash tabasco sauce, if desired
1 teaspoon lemon juice
2 celery stalks (cleaned - but with leaves remaining)

C = 5 P = 2 F = 0

Combine tomato juice, worcestershire sauce, tabasco (if used) and lemon juice. Pour into two tall glasses over ice. Garnish with celery stalks for stirrers and to munch.

*If you desire salt on the rim – take a lemon or lime wedge and run around edge of glass. Dip glass in coarse salt shaking off excess. Then fill as above.

FRUIT MILKSHAKE

Serves 1
Equals
1 Milk Exchange
1 Fruit Exchange
Calories

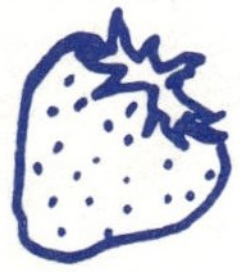

1 ripe peach or nectarine, peeled and chopped or
½ cup raspberries or ¾ cup hulled strawberries
⅓ cup instant non-fat dry milk powder
1 cup ice cubes
2 tablespoons cold water

C = 22 P = 8 F = 0

Blend water and fruit to mix. Add milk powder and ice cubes. Blend until ice melts and drink is rich and frothy. Serve with a straw.

*A drop of almond gives the peach shake a nice flavor.

POPCORN ON A STICK

- great picnic fun -

Cook on a stick - eat from the pouch

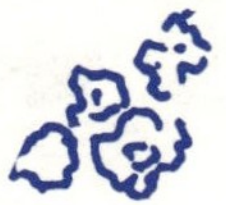

Makes 1 Serving
Equalling
1 Fat Exchange
½ Bread Exchange
82 Calories

1 teaspoon oil
1 tablespoon popcorn, unpopped
salt to taste
1 square heavy aluminum foil 12"

Place oil and unpopped corn in center of foil, twist the edges together to make a loose pouch. Attach pouch to stick with wire, string or folding foil edges together on the stick. Hold over hot coals (or can set on bar-b-que grill). Begin shaking gently as soon as corn starts to pop. When popped, remove from stick, open top of pouch taking care not to be burned on hot escaping steam. Salt to taste and enjoy!

CAMPFIRE POPCORN

Place packet above on grill over hot coals until popped. Remove as soon as finished popping. Carefully open packet allowing steam to escape. Season to taste.

*It's amazing how popcorn cooked outside always tastes great around the campfire, blackened kernels and all!

CAMPFIRE TOASTIES

Makes 20 Toasties
1 Toastie = *35 Calories*
½ Bread Exchange

1 tube (8 ounces) refrigerator biscuits
sticks
hot coals

C = 7.5 P = 1 F = 0

Open biscuits. Cut biscuit dough in half and stretch (like gum) until about 7 inches long. Wrap biscuit around the end of a stick. Slowly roast over fire until biscuit puffs up and browns. These are loads of fun to do and so much safer than sticky marshmallows.

*It's fun to flatten and fill with a bit of cheese or sugar-free jelly before toasting. Be careful. Surprise fillings get **hot.**

FOIL ROASTED CAMP FIRE APPLES

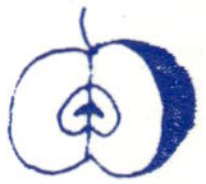

Serves 6
1 Serving Equals
1 Fruit Exchange
1 Fat Exchange
85 Calories

6 small apples
2 tablespoons raisins
1 tablespoon cinnamon or apple pie spice
2 tablespoons butter or margarine

C = 10 P = 0 F = 5

Core apples, cut off collar and scoop out some of the flesh. Place each apple on an individual square of heavy duty aluminum foil. Fill each apple with one teaspoon raisins, ½ teaspoon spice and top with 1 teaspoon butter or margarine. Wrap packages tightly, sealing at the top. Bake on coals approximately 40 minutes until apples are tender.

INDEX

PIES

CAKES AND COOKIES

SPECIAL DESSERTS

TREATS